504

2802

4)

WHY DOCTORS WANT PATIENTS TO READ
RELIEF FROM IBS

"This is the best book written on IBS in the last
ten years. It is very complete and to the point,
making it 'must reading' for doctors to refer to their
patients. I highly recommend it."

"This book gives great insight into and compassion
for a very difficult complex of diseases. The author
. . . documents in great detail how one can not only
cope with irritable bowel syndrome, but become
essentially asymptomatic. I would recommend this
to anyone who had an irritable bowel syndrome or
even thinks he or she has."

Also by Elaine Fantle Shimberg
Published by Ballantine Books:

STROKES: What Families Should Know

RELIEF FROM IBS

Irritable Bowel Syndrome

Elaine Fantle Shimberg

BALLANTINE BOOKS • NEW YORK

Library of Congress Catalog Card Number: 88-30979

ISBN 0-345-36712-X

This edition published by arrangement with M. Evans and Company, Inc.

Printed in Canada

First Ballantine Books Edition: March 1991

To my father
Karl S. Fantle

CONTENTS

PREFACE

Douglas A. Drossman, M.D.
Associate Professor of Medicine and Psychiatry
Division of Digestive Diseases
University of North Carolina School of Medicine
Chapel Hill, N.C. 27514

The irritable bowel syndrome poses difficulties for patients and physicians alike. Although IBS is the most common chronic gastrointestinal disorder in the Western world, IBS sufferers may be reluctant to acknowledge or seek help for their symptoms and, therefore, may lose the prospect of treatment. While IBS is generally a mild and self-limiting condition, a considerable number of patients experience impaired quality of life and work absenteeism and accrue considerable health care costs. Yet funding for research in IBS has a low priority relative to other diseases; therefore our scientific understanding of the disorder and its treatment remains limited. For the family physician and gastroenterologist alike, there is no one diagnostic test: the physician must rely on the history, the physical examination, and a few diagnostic studies to exclude the more serious diseases that may mimic IBS. With no simple test to confirm the diagnosis, some physicians feel uncertain of what they are treating. As a result, they may not acknowledge the syndrome as "real" and may even question the legitimacy of the patient's complaints. This may lead to unneeded tensions in the physician-patient relationship. Finally, there is no one proven treatment, so when the disorder is more refractory, multiple types of therapies may be unsuccessful, leaving both patient and physician feeling frustrated.

While these realities may leave some feeling hopeless and

pessimistic, my experience is that with proper knowledge about the disorder, an understanding physician, and the use of an individualized patient-centered treatment plan, most if not all IBS patients can be helped. In this regard, Ms. Shimberg has made a major contribution toward helping many to achieve this goal.

Being an IBS patient herself, Ms. Shimberg combines her own experience with up-to-date medical information to deliver a concise and practical guide to understanding and managing this perplexing disorder. Through interviews with patients and physicians, we see from a biological, psychological, and social context what it is really like to have IBS. I believe many patients will take solace in knowing they are not alone with their feelings and experiences.

Ms. Shimberg shows the reader in a logical and straightforward fashion how diet, hormonal factors, and the many stresses of daily life can interact with this bowel disorder to produce or worsen symptoms. With this information, she guides the reader toward developing a personalized treatment formulation. I applaud her emphasis on the concept that treatment of IBS involves a partnership: the physician serves as a knowledgeable advisor, while it is the patient who takes primary responsibility for the health care. In my experience, it is when the patient can make the change from passive dependency on the physician toward personal responsibility in the treatment that this illness (or any chronic illness) comes under control.

Ms. Shimberg provides superb insights and suggestions to help the IBS patient accomplish this goal. By using a diary to "track" the symptoms and associated events (a technique I often recommend) the patient may for the first time recognize the inciting factors that aggravate the condition. Then with this new knowledge, Shimberg offers ways to effect lasting behavioral changes, ultimately leading to improvement. Some of her suggestions, such as how to be more efficient and assertive in one's health care, can be generalized to most all phases of daily life.

IBS is a disorder that presents us with a spectrum of symptoms of varying severity, and I believe this book has something to offer for all. Those not in need of medical care will benefit from an improved understanding of the disorder, and will learn of some practical steps to take that will improve their health. For others with more severe symptoms requiring frequent physician visits, the book will not accomplish miracles. As Ms. Shimberg points out, there is no cure, and patients may have chronic or recurrent symptoms for life. But as with all chronic disorders, cure is not the issue: It is the gaining of further knowledge and the development of coping strategies that produce a sense of personal control over the illness and this is the best form of treatment.

FOREWORD

When I sat down to review this book by Elaine Shimberg, I was at first very wary of a book by a layman on irritable bowel syndrome. However, I have found this to be a delightful and in-depth presentation of the subject by an obvious expert: namely, a lady who has the problem.

I feel this book gives great insight into and compassion for a very difficult complex of diseases. The author emphasizes well that organic disease must first be ruled out, but documents in great detail how one, through hard work both on the individual's part as well as that of the physician, can not only cope with irritable bowel syndrome, but become essentially asymptomatic.

I would recommend this to anyone who has an irritable bowel syndrome or even thinks he or she has. It is fun reading, most informative, and certainly worth the reader's time.

Myron Lewis, M.D., FACP, FACG

(Dr. Myron Lewis is a practicing gastroenterologist in Memphis, Tennessee and is president of the American College of Gastroenterology.)

ACKNOWLEDGMENTS

Many people deserve special thanks for sharing both their time and expertise with me. I am especially indebted to Dr. Marvin M. Schuster, Dr. William E. Whitehead, and Dr. Douglas A. Drossman. My thanks and appreciation also to Dr. William Balistreri, Dr. Thomas D. Borkovec, Dr. Joel D. Fyvolent, Sister Judy Lieb, Dr. Robert E. Schaffer, Dr. David Rothman, Belinda Stevenson, and Dr. William R. Carter.

My thanks also to my agent, Herb Katz, for his belief in this project, and to the many people who shared their experiences in dealing with irritable bowel syndrome with me. I have honored their requests to remain anonymous by changing their names as well as merging geographic and career information.

The Holmes-Rahe Social Readjustment Rating Scale was reprinted with permission from the *Journal of Psychosomatic Research II* (1967): 213, Drs. Thomas H. Holmes and R. H. Rahe, Pergamon Journals, Ltd. and from Dr. Thomas H. Holmes.

The table describing the percentage of patients intolerant to particular foods is reprinted with kind permission from Gibson & Jewell: *Topics In Gastroenterology*, Volume 12, Blackwell Scientific Publications.

The quote from Dr. Sidney Cohen was used by permission of *Executive Health Report*, P.O. Box 8880, Chapel Hill, N.C. 27515.

PLEASE NOTE

Before starting your personal search for relief, consult your physician.

The information contained in this book reflects the author's experiences and research and is, in no way, intended to replace professional medical advice. Specific medical opinions can be given to you only by your personal physician who knows you, your unique medical history, your diagnosis, your prognosis, and other relevant data.

THE SYNDROME

An Introduction

You want a conversation stopper? Just tell people you're writing a book about irritable bowel syndrome. Friends and fans (sometimes the same people) ask you to repeat, then say, "Oh . . ." and try to change the subject. Your kids prefer to tell their friends you're working on a trashy novel.

It seems that many people feel comfortable talking about condoms and breast enlargements, watching television ads describing feminine douches and jock itch, and observing what is the nearest thing to simulated sex in movies, but "doo-doo" and "number two" are still conversational no-no holdovers from the nursery.

Television sit-coms and stand-up comics use suggestions of constipation or diarrhea for easy laughs and television ads suggest that most of the world's problems could be cured if only man (and woman) was "regular." Although they are reasonably free discussing sex with others, few people admit, even to their closest friend, that they're concerned about constipation—despite the fact that over 40 million Americans spend more than $225 million on laxatives each year.

But it's time to break the silence, time to talk about irritable bowel syndrome, the "common cold of the intestinal tract" that's plaguing millions, perhaps you, time to let these sufferers know that they're not alone (or crazy) and that there *is* something that can be done.

If you're bright, working hard, pushing fast—and feeling

a debilitating ache in your gut that comes and goes—you may be one of the more than 22 million Americans, most of them women, suffering symptoms that are *not* life-threatening and *can* be relieved.

Cramps, fatigue, gas pains that can be so severe they attack your lower back, diarrhea alternating with constipation—symptoms that attack you on the job, on vacation, and on a date—*can* be controlled, *can* be relieved entirely.

For terrific people who want to feel terrific, here's a book I produced the hard way. I was a victim of IBS until I learned how not to be. I'd like to share that information with you.

"You're writing a book about irritable bowel syndrome?" My friend, Kathy (not her real name), wrinkled her nose in disgust. "Why not write about something we can talk about!"

Yet, just five minutes later, Kathy *was* talking about irritable bowel syndrome, telling me how she coped with the problems it created in *her* life.

A top account executive with a Chicago public relations firm, Kathy described how gas pains often disrupted her right in the middle of a presentation to important clients; how the sensation of impending diarrhea once caused her to leave the head table at a professional seminar just before she was about to be introduced as the keynote speaker; and how she "cased" restaurants before entertaining clients there.

"I need to know where the ladies' room is," she explained, "just in case I have to make a mad dash."

She had become "bathroom bound," obsessively making mental notes of toilet facility locations in office buildings, airports, and department stores. At times, her symptoms created so much anxiety and discomfort and so greatly interfered with her work and the image she was trying to convey—that of a highly skilled and effective executive—that she considered quitting her job.

No, she had not seen a doctor lately. Two years ago, her internist had told her she was "just nervous—highly strung." She was embarrassed to return with the same complaints. Nevertheless, her symptoms persisted and she felt depressed.

I was most sympathetic. I, too, suffer from IBS, the "common cold of the intestinal tract." But Kathy and I are hardly unique. IBS is a chronic disorder of the colon, afflicting an estimated 17 percent of the adult population of our country alone.

Although it is not life-threatening, IBS can be severe and even debilitating, interfering with job, social life, and other activities. It's a major cause of work absenteeism in the United States, second only to the common cold. Even to those with mild symptoms, IBS can be unpleasant and annoying. It affects all age groups, but particularly adults between the ages of twenty and fifty—two females for every male. Clearly, Kathy and I fit the profile.

Looking back, I realized that my intestinal tract has always been my "weak spot." As a youngster, it acted up the night before the opening session of school, backstage before the curtain on a community theater play, or when I was fatigued. "Just nerves," I was told. "Learn to live with it."

As an adult—a full-time writer, mother of five, and wife of a real estate developer and theatrical producer—I never had time to be sick. Yet occasionally, and often inconveniently, I did feel intestinal discomfort. It ranged from slight pain—just a vague annoyance—to prolonged periods of constipation or severe diarrhea which sometimes became debilitating.

Although I could never pin down any particular offending food, I had the vague feeling that there were certain foods that sometimes "bothered" me. But just when I thought I had identified one or more foods to avoid, I ended up eating them with no trace of discomfort.

When the pains continued to crop up for no apparent reason and with no traceable pattern, I harbored the conviction that I must have colon cancer, ulcerative colitis, or some other serious disease. As a medical writer, I have a library filled with medical books. In no time, I had come up with a myriad of possible diseases that somewhat fit my symptoms.

No stranger to research, I tried to pin down the cause of my symptoms. Was it something I ate or drank? No, not always. Did the symptoms arise when I was tired? Only at times. Could it be tension? Often, but not specially so.

Then I did what I should have done in the beginning. I went to my internist, who examined me carefully and found me to be in perfect health. "It's 'spastic colon.' You'll have to learn to live with it," he said, and referred me to a specialist when I asked for a second opinion.

I consulted a gastroenterologist (a physician who specializes in diseases of the stomach and intestines). He examined me, took barium X rays of my stomach and intestines, examined me visually with a sigmoidoscope, and checked stool samples to rule out cancer and other potentially dangerous diseases. He pronounced me to be healthy.

"It's irritable bowel syndrome," he said. "You'll have to learn to live with it."

I saw a nutritionist who questioned me about my diet. She said I ate well-balanced meals (for the most part) and suggested I eat a little more fiber.

"You're healthy," she said. "You've got 'mucous colitis.' You'll have to learn to live with it."

I even got a fortune cookie that told me I was "strong in body and spirit and would enjoy life." It gave me no diagnosis and said nothing about having to "learn to live with it."

Obviously, I was thankful to have "nothing serious." Nevertheless, I continued—on occasion and for no specific reason I could pinpoint—to suffer from bothersome symptoms. The fact that I was not alone in my discomfort, and that I did, indeed, have millions of fellow sufferers, was of little solace.

A 1980 study of apparently healthy people showed that "up to one third of subjects from the general population have been found to have symptoms associated with irritable bowel syndrome."[1] Also known as "irritable colon," "spastic colon," "nervous diarrhea," and "mucous colitis,'' IBS is an especially difficult disorder because doctors don't know exactly what causes it. A combination of different factors trigger it in each person, and the treatment varies according to the individual and his or her unique body makeup.

Many physicians who deal with irritable bowel syndrome admit to often feeling frustrated when dealing with IBS patients because it's hard to treat this disease. It's a chronic condition; it cannot be cured. Something may seem to work one time, but not another. Patients, in turn, may sense this frustration and translate it to mean either, ''The doctor thinks it's all in my head,'' or ''The doctor's angry with me because I still feel rotten.''

Actually, until quite recently, many doctors did feel that irritable bowel syndrome was a psychosomatic disorder. When all the tests and X rays turned up negative and yet the patient continued to complain of diarrhea, constipation, or a combination of both, the next doctor on the referral list often was a psychiatrist.

Unfortunately, there still are doctors today who feel that there is no medical basis for the complaints of IBS symptoms. ''If it doesn't show up on tests, it must be mental,'' they feel, and they pack the patient off to get his or her head checked. Naturally, this tends to create more stress in a patient who already has been suffering very real pains and very real diarrhea and constipation.

Some physicians don't seem to be aware of irritable bowel syndrome and tend to consider almost every other diagnosis first. Carol, a lobbyist in Chicago, went to see her gynecologist after suffering from extremely bad low stomach pains for two weeks.

''I would have thought it was my appendix,'' she said, ''but I had that removed when I was eleven. The gynecologist thought I had an ovarian cyst and suggested rest. I canceled my scheduled vacation and sat home, worrying that maybe I had an inflammatory pelvic disease.

''I returned to the doctor for another pelvic examination. I think I had even greater pain from the exam than I was having before. He then decided I probably had a urinary tract infection and prescribed antibiotics. The pain grew worse. I really couldn't move. The doctor suggested exploratory surgery. I really panicked and went for another opinion.

"I saw a general internist. He said I was a 'very tense young woman.' I remember snarling at him that if he had been in as much pain as I was, he'd be tense, too. He ran a series of tests, including barium X rays of the upper and lower gastrointestinal tract. When nothing bad showed up on any of the tests, he said I had irritable bowel syndrome and gave me some muscle relaxants and some hints on how to relax. I had missed three weeks of work and was convinced I was crazy. Instead, it was irritable bowel syndrome."

Although certain factors may trigger IBS—diet, stress, and hormones are the major ones—the particular interaction among foods, stress, hormones, and fatigue often differs between individuals and even within the same individual. (See Illustration A.)

For example, while each sufferer quickly learns the importance of maintaining adequate fiber in the diet, adding more bulk is not always the "quick solution." Indeed, for some IBS patients, additional bulk may intensify the very symptoms it is intended to lessen.

For this reason, treatment of IBS becomes extremely personalized. And here the patient must become an active participant. Please note that this is NOT to say that a person should self-diagnose him- or herself. The first step is *always* to seek professional medical advice. But once medical expertise has ruled out other disease possibilities and the physician has made the diagnosis of "irritable bowel syndrome," the patient becomes the detective, using the guidelines set out by the doctor to solve the mystery, what triggers IBS in *me* and how can I control it?

This is difficult for many of us. We expect to hear our doctor say, "This is what is wrong with you. This is what you need to do to correct the problem." We often feel short-changed if we are not handed a prescription for a drug to make everything "all better."

ILLUSTRATION A

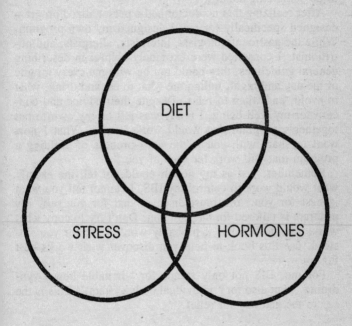

FACTORS RELATING TO IBS

But doctors cannot cure IBS. It is a chronic condition, which means that once you have it, you have it for good. No medicine or magic wand can make it go away for always. But you can learn to control IBS, to find relief from its troublesome symptoms. I did.

A few years ago I reached a decision. I was no longer willing to "learn to live with it." Instead, I was determined to do something about it.

After realizing that no doctor had a personalized program designed specifically for *me*, I designed my own program. While the gastroenterologists, internists, allergists, and nutritionists I consulted were extremely helpful in describing general guidelines, they could not be with me every minute of the day and night, telling me what to eat and drink, what to avoid, and when to relax. Despite their advice and concern for my well-being, I really was left on my own to put together a program that would work for me. What I now want to share with you is the very process of building a program that will work for each of you.

Remember, just as my doctor could not tell me exactly what would work to control my IBS, I cannot tell you what is best for you. You must discover that for yourself. *My* program is tailored for *me*, not you. Don't try to copy what works for me because it probably won't work for you; instead, use this book to help you discover what works best for *you*.

For me, IBS not only stands for "irritable bowel syndrome," but also for "individual body system." This is the *key* to the gateway for relief.

2

Where is Your Colon?

"Do you know where your colon is?" sounds something like the message that comes on just before the late evening news and asks the same thing about your children. Unfortunately, for many people, the answer to both questions is no.

I posed the question concerning the colon's location, very unscientifically, to twenty people in a busy shopping mall. The question was presented as part of a survey being taken for a medical writer. Other less threatening questions included: "Have you seen a doctor in the last year?" "Are there any foods you are unable to eat? If so, which ones?" And, coming after the "colon question," "Have you ever heard of irritable bowel syndrome?"

Most of those who stopped to listen to my questions looked uneasy, as though it was a pop quiz no one had told them about. Three of the twenty walked away without answering the "colon question" at all, although they had been cooperative with the first two.

Among the seventeen who did remain to tackle the last two questions, the answers varied widely, ranging from, "I can't believe you're asking me that. How should I know?" to "I . . . uh . . . I think it's somewhere around the butt."

Another, who said she thought she had IBS, said she thought the colon was "somewhere above the stomach." Others placed it "in the stomach," "in the back," "in the gut," or as "part of the digestive system." A graduate student shrugged and grinned. "The only colon I can think of is on term papers and I think it goes inside the quotation marks."

Many of the people just wrinkled their foreheads, stared at the ceiling, and may still be thinking about it.

I've asked the question of others, especially those who do suffer from irritable bowel syndrome. Although many people know they have a colon and acknowledge that it's involved in some way with the hurt they're feeling, they can't locate it exactly. Just as many of us received little formal instruction in geography and still can't place countries, rivers, or mountains, we also have scant information about the map of our own body. Memories of junior high health class reveal only faded thoughts of poorly made *You're Growing Up* movies, adolescent embarrassment, and the sense of haste to get on with what seemed like more important issues—how to sink a free throw or spike a volleyball.

What is the digestive tract?

While I have no desire to make this a book about the digestive system—it would take an entire book to fully describe this fascinating and complex process that fuels our body—I do think a brief description might be useful.

To put it in its most simple form, our digestive system works a great deal like the early "Betsy Wetsy" dolls. Little girls, myself included, used to spend hours holding miniature glass baby bottles filled with water to a hole in our rubber doll's lips only to marvel at the fact that, seconds later, the cloth diaper at the other end was wet.

Our own digestive tract is not too dissimilar to the doll's "something in—something out" tube system. Also tube-like, our digestive system runs from one end of our body to the other, a distance of some forty feet, from the mouth to the anus. Fortunately, unlike the rubber doll whose tract I clogged with a spoonful of oatmeal which hardened like plaster and totally put her out of commission, we also have digestive glands which help us break down the food taken in so it can be absorbed and used by our body.

How does it work?

Food enters the mouth where it is chewed by the teeth, stirred by the tongue, and mixed with saliva, which begins the chemical action necessary to break up the starches. The food then is forced to the back of the mouth, where it is swallowed and forced down into another part of the tube, the ten-inch esophagus, or second section of the digestive tract. Special muscles force the food from there into the stomach, where the food is battered and churned into small pieces and worked on by various digestive chemicals. The stomach is protected from digesting itself by special mucus secretions on its walls.

From the stomach, the near-liquid mixture of food and digestive juices (called *chyme*) passes into the duodenum, the upper part of the about twenty-foot-long small intestine. More chemicals are secreted by various glands to help in the digestive process. Food is pushed along by muscle contractions in the intestine known as "peristalsis."

It is while in the small intestine that the food is completely digested by pancreatic juices, intestinal juices, and bile. Nutrients are absorbed through the walls of the small intestine and into the bloodstream to help the body restore itself and maintain its energy level.

Like sludge in a sewer system, the remaining undigested matter moves into the "drying tank," the approximately five-foot-long large intestine, or colon, where much of the water portion is absorbed back into the body. It is here in the colon where pain and discomfort begin for those suffering from irritable bowel syndrome. For them, the normal rhythmic action of the colon goes out of sync, causing pain, distention, diarrhea, constipation, or alternating diarrhea and constipation.

For most people, however, the colon does its work effectively and efficiently, without drawing much attention to itself. The remaining waste—undigested bits of seed and fiber, bacteria, small amounts of salt and bile, and water—passes into the rectum and is eliminated as a bowel movement at the end section of the digestive tract, through the anus.

Why is it necessary to know all this?

Most of us feel a little insecure about taking our car to the repair shop. There's really no reason. It's our car, we know its funny little quirks better than a stranger does, and we know it isn't working the way it should. Why do we hate going in to Friendly Eddie's Car Repair? Probably because we really know so little about our car. We don't have the proper vocabulary to explain what's wrong and often that makes it difficult to communicate the problem. We're afraid Friendly Eddie is going to run a lot of expensive tests in order to see why the gizmo is making a "barking" sound or the "whatchamacallit" is clicking.

Seeing our doctor is the same, and more so. Usually, when we see the doctor we're sick or hurting. In addition to being time-consuming and expensive, the tests often are uncomfortable and sometimes downright painful. When we lack the proper vocabulary for body parts or we're self-conscious about talking about them, it makes it difficult to convey our message to the doctor. We feel embarrassed.

"It hurts 'down there,' " an older woman told her doctor. He sensed she wasn't talking about her ankle, but it took him a great deal of valuable time—an asset in short supply in most physicians' offices—for him to figure out through gentle questioning whether she meant she had pain in her rectum, vagina, uterus, or intestinal tract.

Knowing where things are in your body as well as what to call them is especially important when you have irritable bowel syndrome. As IBS is a functional disorder, nothing shows up on X rays, sigmoidoscope, or in other tests. The physician must make the diagnosis based on what he or she *doesn't* find on the tests and on your description of how you feel and what happens to you.

What can go wrong?

When all of the digestive processes work as they should, you should be unaware of most of the activity and, fortunately, can take digestion and eliminating rather matter-of-factly. But we are not rubber dolls, passively taking in food at one end and expelling it at another. The miraculous digestive system can be thrown off in all of us by a myriad of things, from drugs or stress to infection and disease. When there are problems, as there are with those suffering from irritable bowel syndrome, you quickly become all too painfully aware that something is wrong with your digestive system. And it is.

3

What Is IBS? How Did I Get It? What Can I Do About It?

If you're one of the approximately 22 million Americans suffering from irritable bowel syndrome, it probably is of great, but not total, comfort to know that IBS is not a "serious" disorder. It does not predispose you to other chronic or life-threatening diseases such as cancer or ulcerative colitis. It will not get worse. You do not require surgery. It is not life threatening. People don't die from IBS.

What are the symptoms?

Unfortunately, you often may feel as though you could die. The symptoms—gas, stomach pain, bowel dysfunction with alternating constipation and diarrhea—frequently leave you exhausted, frustrated, and uneasy about distancing yourself too far from the bathroom. It can affect your work, your social life, your leisure time, and actually dominate your entire life-style. It's no wonder that those suffering from IBS often become both anxious and depressed.

IBS is a chronic disorder, accounting for 40 to 70 percent of all gastrointestinal referrals and for 25 percent of a gastroenterologist's practice.[1] In addition to abdominal pain with constipation, diarrhea, or alternating constipation and diarrhea, its symptoms may include:

- abdominal distension
- relief of pain by a bowel movement

- looser bowel movements with pain onset
- more frequent bowel movements with pain onset
- mucus in the stool
- a sense of incomplete evacuation[2]

A 1984 study by W. Grant Thompson, M.D., chief of the Division of Gastroenterology at the Ottawa Civic Hospital in Canada, revealed that 99 percent of those with IBS have at least two of these symptoms. In addition, some people experience gas, nausea, and heartburn. The symptoms tend to seesaw between mild and severe for no apparent reason and then disappear even more mysteriously. Although a patient may be symptom-free for several years, recurrence is the rule. According to Marvin M. Schuster, M.D., professor of medicine and psychiatry at Johns Hopkins University School of Medicine and chief of the Division of Digestive Diseases at Francis Scott Key Medical Center in Baltimore, "Symptoms vary from patient to patient, but are consistent for a given patient, although severity may fluctuate."

For most people, IBS symptoms begin in late adolescence, although IBS can and does show up in children (see Chapter 20). In the United States, women are twice as likely to suffer from IBS as men. These figures, however, may reflect the fact that in America, women are more likely to seek medical attention than men. In India, according to Douglas A. Drossman, M.D., associate professor of medicine and psychiatry in the Division of Digestive Diseases and Nutrition at the University of North Carolina School of Medicine in Chapel Hill, the sex ratio is reversed. There the ratio is two to one, men over women. This may be related to economic or cultural differences; men tend to go to physicians more than women do in India, whereas in Western cultures, women go to the doctor more for these types of problems.

Irritable bowel syndrome is considered to be a young person's disease, with at least half the patients seen before their thirty-fifth birthdays. When someone older is diagnosed, they usually have had symptoms off and on since childhood. In fact, symptoms that begin in older people who have had no history of intestinal problems in childhood, adolescence, or early adulthood may reflect something other than IBS.

While symptoms usually include stomach pain, bloating, gas, constipation, diarrhea, or a combination of constipation and diarrhea, they can and do vary. Some IBS sufferers have mild pain, some constipation, and no diarrhea; others have severe abdominal pain, constipation, and then diarrhea; still others may experience no pain but have diarrhea—especially immediately following breakfast—every day.

Dr. Marvin M. Schuster says, "The pain is most often experienced in the lower abdomen, usually in the left lower quadrant, but its location varies from one person to another as does its quality, which may be described as being cramplike, steady, dull, sharp, or burning."

NOTE: While these are the symptoms of irritable bowel syndrome, they also could be those of more serious disorders. Only your physician can determine whether your symptoms are caused by irritable bowel syndrome or something else by taking a careful medical history, performing a complete physical examination, and running various laboratory tests. Never try to diagnose yourself! Since many serious diseases have similar symptoms to those of IBS, your doctor must rule these out. Always seek proper medical care!

It is not in your head

Irritable bowel syndrome is considered to be a "functional" disorder. That means that no sign of the disorder can be determined through the use of X rays, sigmoidoscopes, or other diagnostic techniques. But IBS is *not* an emotional disorder. No matter what you may have been told, it is not "all in your mind." The problem is in your colon, not your head.

Dr. Douglas A. Drossman puts it simply: "IBS is the gut's response to the environment." That includes dietary factors, hormonal changes, family habits, and stress levels.

Although stress and emotional upsets can and often do trigger IBS, they are not the primary cause.

Researchers have discovered that people who suffer from IBS have abnormal movement patterns in their colon, caused by a hyperactive enteric nervous system, the nervous system that controls the intestine. They experience excessive movement or spasms in this section of the digestive tract, which connects the small intestine to the anus (see Illustration B).

No food is digested in the colon. That work is done very efficiently by the small intestine. The function of the colon is to absorb water and salts from digestive products that enter from the small intestine, therefore acting as a type of "drying tank." When a spasm occurs, the cramping can trap stool in much the same way a kink in a plastic hose traps water. This produces constipation. When a bowel movement does take place, it is with difficulty, through straining, and the stool is hard and said to resemble "rabbit pellets" or "rocklike marbles," or is described as "pencil-thin" or "ribbonlike."

What is constipation?

Constipation and the fear of constipation is a major concern of millions of otherwise healthy people. While it can become a real problem for the elderly and bedridden, who may suffer from fecal impaction (where the stool becomes so tightly packed in the bowel that it can't be expelled normally), it usually is no more than a source of discomfort to those who suffer from it. Unfortunately, part of the problem in dealing with constipation is a lack of specific criteria for determining what really constitutes constipation. Most physicians define it as having at least three days between bowel movements and then having hard dry stools that are difficult to pass.

But many people think they suffer from constipation any time they don't have a daily bowel movement. Actually, there is a wide range of what is considered "normal." For some people, "normal" is three times a day; for others, it

ILLUSTRATION B

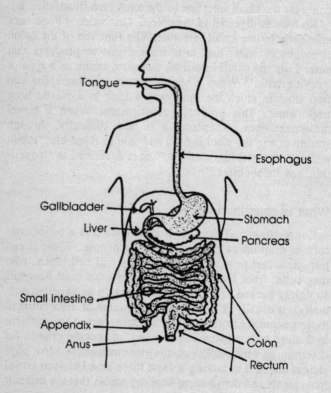

Tongue

Esophagus

Gallbladder

Liver

Stomach

Pancreas

Small intestine

Appendix

Anus

Colon

Rectum

may be three times a week! It's important to know what constitutes "normal" for you.

Constipation is caused by many different conditions ranging from the imaginary (thinking you're constipated because you missed a day without moving your bowels) to poor diet or various medications or serious diseases. Usually, however, constipation is due to nothing more than:

- a lack of adequate fiber in the diet
- inadequate liquid intake, especially water
- insufficient exercise
- ignoring the urge to defecate
- dependence on laxatives
- tension
- hormonal changes, such as those preceding menstruation
- certain drugs and antidepressant medications, such as high blood pressure medicine, painkillers containing codeine, and antacids containing aluminum compounds

One woman traced her problems with constipation to her childhood and the elementary school she attended. "The bathrooms were in the basement," she said. "You had to raise your hand to be excused, get a pass, and then walk downstairs into this dark and somewhat musty basement area. There was no way I was going to do any of that. It was too traumatic. Instead, I got used to just putting it off. To this day, I won't use public toilets. When I travel, I'm constipated for days!" Many women shared similar memories and confessed to feeling uncomfortable or unable to use public toilet facilities.

There are, of course, medical conditions such as pregnancy, hormonal imbalances, hemorrhoids, and cancer that can cause constipation, so it's always best to consult your physician if you're having problems or even think you are. Be sure to give *your* definition of constipation so your doctor knows what you consider it to be. But once you've been reassured that it's nothing serious and not to worry, take that advice—and stop taking laxatives or enemas to make yourself "regular."

Instead, help your colon by:

• increasing fiber in your diet
• increasing fluid intake, preferably water
• increasing physical movement
• scheduling a regular time (usually after breakfast) to move your bowels
• relaxing when you feel yourself tensing

These and other suggestions will be dealt with in more depth in the fourth section of this book, entitled "Treating."

What is diarrhea?

Almost everyone has suffered from diarrhea—loose and frequent bowel movements—at some time. It might result from an intestinal upset caused by either a virus or a bacterial infection. It can also result from prescription drugs, such as antibiotics or over-the-counter remedies like laxatives, aspirin, certain antacids, and iron pills (iron pills also turn the stool black).

The condition called diarrhea—an abnormally frequent discharge of more or less fluid fecal matter from the bowel—can also occur as the result of eating too much fruit, emotional stress, intestinal parasites, lactose intolerance, food poisoning, or traveling to another country and drinking water or eating food that contains bacteria or parasites upsetting to your intestinal tract.

There are also serious conditions that can cause diarrhea, so, once again, you need to consult your physician if it lasts for more than a few days. Be sure to describe what you call diarrhea as there is no specific agreed-on medical definition. Remember, too, that dehydration is always a possibility when diarrhea is prolonged, so be sure to drink plenty of liquids—preferably water—if you have diarrhea.

IBS sufferers have alternating diarrhea and constipation

Unfortunately, IBS sufferers usually experience the frustration of having *both* constipation and diarrhea, although many tend more to one than the other. Irritable bowel syndrome is a bowel motility (movement) disorder. When there are spasms in the colon, the movement forces stool to move too quickly, before the fluid part of the feces can be absorbed. This leads to diarrhea.

Occasionally, there also will be mucus in the stool. For this reason, IBS often is called "mucous colitis." The term is incorrect, however, because "colitis" refers to an inflammation of the large bowel, and with irritable bowel syndrome there is no sign of any inflammation anywhere in the digestive tract. The presence of mucus is caused by the increased motility or activity in the colon. It is *not* a sign of infection or disease.

Although diarrhea usually occurs in IBS sufferers immediately after eating breakfast, it can appear after other meals or at any other (often inconvenient) time throughout the day. Food itself doesn't trigger the explosive diarrhea, but instead activates the gastrocolic reflex, a neurological and chemical response which tells the colon to empty itself.

Interestingly, people with irritable bowel syndrome are seldom awakened from sleep with the feeling of impending diarrhea. This does happen to those suffering from serious colon diseases such as ulcerative colitis or Crohn's disease, however, and is important information to share with your doctor.

Also tell your doctor immediately if you experience any blood in your stool. Although it *may* be caused by hemorrhoids, bleeding is not usual with IBS and should always be checked out by your physician.

The symptoms of IBS *do* mimic many other stomach and intestinal disorders. As the symptoms vary from person to person, you can't determine what *you* have from what the doctor told your cousin. Always check with your physician!

Why me?

Medical experts really don't know why certain people have irritable bowel syndrome and others don't. It may just be the toss of the coin—your Achilles' heel may be your colon, just as migraine sufferers get headaches and asthma patients wheeze. Both afflictions, as with IBS, have medical causes, but are exacerbated by stress and emotions.

Most physicians dealing with irritable bowel syndrome agree that there is no "IBS personality," as such. There are no unique personality characteristics or patterns that are peculiar to IBS patients. Yet according to William E. Whitehead, Ph.D., of the Department of Psychiatry at Johns Hopkins University School of Medicine and the Division of Digestive Diseases at Francis Scott Key Medical Center in Baltimore, many IBS patients reported that they had numerous colds as children and received toys or "treatfoods" when they were ill. He suggests that children with "RAP" (recurrent abdominal pain) might be modeling or unconsciously copying their parents' behavior. That is, the parents may have complained of stomach pains, constipation, or diarrhea, and the children copied the response from them.

Some researchers feel that childhood deprivation—real or imagined—plays some part in making one susceptible to IBS. In an Australian study, 333 consecutive patients with irritable bowel syndrome were interviewed and their childhood psychosocial environments examined. By the age of fifteen, 31 percent of the patients had lost a parent through death, divorce, or separation; 19 percent had an alcoholic parent; and 61 percent reported unsatisfactory relationships with, or between, their parents.[3] The important influence of childhood deprivation in the etiology (study of causes) of IBS is supported by these findings.

But there are also actual documented physical differences between those with IBS and those without. Studies by many researchers reveal that people with IBS tend to have lower colon pain tolerance and to report colon pain sooner than control groups without IBS. IBS sufferers *do* have a different motor response. But that is only in regard to gut pain.

When Dr. Marvin M. Schuster compared IBS patients' reactions to pain with those of non-IBS volunteers by holding their hands in ice water, he discovered that the IBS volunteers had a *higher* tolerance for ice-water-inflicted pain than the control group (i.e., those volunteers without IBS). Clearly, the weakness is in the colon, not in the individual's overall reaction to pain and discomfort.

But if, as numerous health surveys indicate, 17 percent of the general population suffers from IBS symptoms, something drives certain IBS sufferers and not others to see a doctor. It may be that individuals who seek medical help feel pain more intensely. They may be suffering from more stress or may have more need for a doctor's care. For many, unfortunately, it is not the first time they have seen a doctor for stomach-related problems. It is not uncommon to hear of IBS sufferers whose bodies bear scars from appendectomies or gallbladder surgery. Many of the female patients have had hysterectomies as well.

What can be done about IBS?

Dr. Marvin Schuster lists four major points for IBS sufferers to remember:

1. Don't self-diagnose. *Always* seek professional medical advice to rule out serious problems.
2. If you receive the diagnosis of IBS from your doctor, don't confuse it with ulcerative colitis. The latter is a serious colon disease characterized by inflammation of the lining of the colon. There is no inflammation with IBS. Ulcerative colitis differs greatly from IBS in both treatment and prognosis.
3. Remember that the problem is in the colon, not in your mind. You have a very real abnormality in the nervous system that serves your intestines. While it's true that stress and emotional factors often trigger an attack, they are *not* the primary cause.
4. Once your doctor has made the diagnosis of IBS—and you've received a second opinion, if you desire—stop

seeing doctors. Don't keep "shopping around" for a doctor who can cure you or who will agree to perform surgery because you keep hounding him or her to do something.

According to Dr. Ernie Chaney, associate professor of family medicine at the University of Kansas School of Medicine, "The emotional and economical cost of 'doctor hopping' is not limited to needless office consultations. It also involves unnecessary testing. Patients who have had three barium enemas in a year, along with other tests, are sometimes referred to a subspecialist who tests them all over again."[4]

IBS is a chronic disease; that means that although it may be dormant for a while, you will have episodic flare-ups—usually when you're under pressure and have little time or patience for feeling badly.

It's important to have a physician you feel comfortable with and one who is familiar with you as an individual and with your particular problems. Each person with IBS is different. Accept that irritable bowel syndrome is a chronic disease and begin to try to figure out how you can best control its symptoms.

And that latter point, of course, is what this book is all about—learning what works best for you, personally, to control the painful, bothersome, and frustrating symptoms of IBS.

Each of us is unique

The miracle of life encompasses the fact that each of us—even siblings born to the same parents—is unique. Not only do we have distinctive fingerprints, but we also react to stimuli in different ways. Some of our reactions are learned responses, of course. We often respond as we were taught—silently or verbally—by our parents. But even within one family, there may be those with tranquil personalities and those who flare at the slightest provocation.

We also react differently internally. One child may be the

"billy goat" of the family, able to digest anything but tin cans, while a sibling may grow queasy just by looking at a television commercial promoting a particular brand of cooking oil.

While patients with irritable bowel syndrome do have abnormal, exaggerated contractions in their colon, what specifically triggers IBS is more than just a faulty intestinal tract. It's what Dr. Douglas A. Drossman calls "the gut's reaction to the environment." It is a combination of causes, and this combination varies from person to person, even within a family.

We all react differently to food combinations, for example, depending on allergies, emotional reactions the food groupings evoke, medicines we may be taking, childhood memories, or other factors. Making it even more difficult to pin down specifics is that each person may react differently to stimuli depending on what else is going on in his or her life at the time.

Irritable bowel syndrome is a continuum disease, more bothersome to some than to others and varying in severity on different occasions. It is *your* problem, however, not your doctor's, and regardless of how sympathetic and understanding a physician may be, in the long run, it is your disorder and you must take an active role in treating it.

The remaining chapters of this book are divided into three major sections: Triggering, Tracking, and Treating.

By working with your physician and applying the principles found in the following pages, you should be able to learn what triggers irritable bowel syndrome in *you* and to develop a personal program for relief from IBS.

= TRIGGERING =

===== **4** =====

Stress and Emotional Factors

Although IBS is a physical disorder—caused by increased movement in the colon—there is little doubt that it is often triggered and made worse by stress and emotional factors, as well as other factors such as diet and hormones.

Obviously, no one lives without encountering stressful situations. You can hardly wrap yourself in cotton wadding and plastic bubble paper and hide out in a cave. And even if you could, you'd soon experience stress from being cold, hungry, and afraid a bear would find you. As the late stress researcher and expert Dr. Hans Selye said, "Complete freedom from stress is death."

Stress can be "good" or "bad"

Stress in and of itself isn't a bad thing. Actually, many stressful situations also bring us great joy and satisfaction— such as taking part in athletic competitions, traveling, performing artistically, or being reunited with a loved one. There are other events, however, that can create extreme and harmful stress—such as being surrounded by urban noise pollution, being constantly interrupted by the telephone, being kept awake by your neighbor's barking dog, working in a smoke-filled office or facing glare from computer screens or improper lighting, being deadlocked by frustrating and boring work, or finding yourself crushed by time pressures.

The triggering event doesn't even have to be real to be stressful. An imagined fear or concern can be every bit as stressful as if it were actual. Someone worrying that his or her job is on the line, or that a mate is straying or ill, or fantasizing "the worst" happening any minute, can experience real stress and its resulting negative effects.

Some people spend much of their time, unproductively, worrying about things that never happen. (Actually, worrying about things that *do* happen isn't very productive either. It only takes the place of action.) These habitual worriers build up complex scenarios, stacked on a foundation of fantasy, that teeter precariously on top of one another.

According to Dr. William R. Carter, professor of clinical psychology in the Department of Behavioral Medicine and Psychology at the University of Virginia School of Medicine, 15 percent of our population are chronic worriers. He and other psychologists, former members of a research team at Pennsylvania State University, studied worrying and worriers. They concluded that worrying doesn't help solve problems. Actually, it interferes with one's thought processes and the effectiveness of the activity at hand. It creates additional stress. And since stress triggers IBS symptoms, additional stress is just what we who suffer from irritable bowel syndrome do *not* need.

But it's no good just telling yourself to stop worrying. The late Hans Selye wrote, "You must find something to put in place of the worrying thoughts to chase them away."[1] Although that may seem simple enough advice, it's often very hard to put into practice. Sometimes it involves reexamining your value system. You may have to ask yourself why you worry and what you gain from it before you're able to banish worrying to the attic. Many of the chapters in the "Treating" section of this book describe ways in which you can chase those worrying thoughts away by substituting more positive action.

Studies suggest that "IBS patients have been exposed to more stressful events than have normal subjects" and that they also "worry or become anxious in response to relatively minor and everyday concerns, as well as being exposed more frequently to major stressors."[2]

While the cause and level of stress varies from person to person—you may feel comfortable and enthusiastic at the prospect of walking into a room filled with strangers; I feel anxious and tense at large gatherings—most of us typically do experience stress to some degree in certain similar situations, such as flying in a plane in turbulent weather, giving a speech when you don't feel totally prepared, being robbed, or being caught in traffic that makes you late for an important appointment.

Anxiety, intestinal distress, and diarrhea are common reactions to these situations, whether you have IBS or not. In fact, in one study, 70 percent of the "normal" (that is, nonpatient) population surveyed reported that they suffered from changes in bowel function in reaction to stressful situations. Over half of this group also experienced stomach pain under stress.[3]

But those who suffer from irritable bowel syndrome seem to suffer more. Their symptoms tend to be triggered by events that other people seem to be able either to take in stride or to react to in other physical ways, such as by getting headaches, stiff necks, or having asthma attacks. For those with IBS, the gut is the target area.

IBS sufferers have lower stress tolerances

Studies suggest that irritable bowel syndrome sufferers tend to have lower stress tolerance levels than non-IBS patients. Things "get" to you more and they get you in the gut, your body's weak spot. It's possible that this reaction may be a conditioned or learned response dating from your childhood. Perhaps you had frequent stomachaches as a youngster and often were allowed to stay home from school because of them. Your parents might have fussed over you more when you were sick, bringing you meals on a tray in bed, preparing special "treat" foods, or surprising you with little gifts to "make you feel better."

You also may have sensed or actually experienced great

parental concern about your bowel habits. A female marketing executive, now suffering from frequent episodes of IBS, recalled being given laxatives and enemas as a child whenever she missed having a daily bowel movement.

"I longed for a morning kiss when I came down for breakfast," she said. "Instead, I got quizzed on the state of my bowels."

In a recent study in North Carolina of three groups—patients with IBS, nonpatients (people who have not visited a doctor) with IBS symptoms, and people with no symptoms—"more patients, and in most cases nonpatients with IBS, reported poorer general health and headaches, stomachaches, and bowel complaints during childhood . . . Loss and separation during childhood and in the current family, and conflicted or dependent maternal relationships were also more frequently reported among patients and nonpatients."[4]

The above study certainly adds validity to the thought that stress—especially stress occurring in childhood, before the individual has acquired sufficient coping techniques—could influence the development of IBS in individuals with that tendency. While that knowledge may be of little value to you now as an adult who does suffer from irritable bowel syndrome, if you are a parent, it may help you to reexamine your attitudes and behaviors toward illness and assist you in teaching stress reduction techniques to your children.

Stress can make you sick

This is not to say that IBS is all in your head. The physical problem—increased motility—is in your colon and is very real. But this increased movement can, and often does, react to stress and emotion. These findings are far from new. Physicians have known for a long time that there was a strong interrelationship between emotions and one's physical condition.

In 1822, doctors had the rare opportunity to observe firsthand how the stomach digests food when a Canadian fur trapper was accidentally shot. The injury left a two-and-a-half-inch hole in his stomach. For eight years the attending physician, an American named William Beaumont, studied how digestive juices work on food and monitored changes in the stomach lining as the trapper's emotions changed.

In 1902, American physiologist Walter B. Cannon noted a cessation in bowel activity in cats who were frightened by a growling dog.[5]

Early in the 1900s, the great Russian physiologist Ivan Petrovich Pavlov discovered that strong emotion could trigger gastrointestinal activity by increasing the flow of digestive juices in the stomach.

The study of the intertwining of emotions, stress, and one's physical well-being has continued well into the twentieth century. In 1949, Drs. T. P. Almy, F. Kern, Jr., and M. Tulin performed a fascinating and telling experiment with a fourth year medical student.[6] The subject was told only that the experiment would require preliminary proctoscopy (inspection of the interior of the colon through the use of a special instrument inserted rectally).

After ten minutes of observation, during which the bowel was relaxed, the student was told that the doctors had discovered a rectal cancer and the doctors wanted permission to perform a biopsy. In the following twenty minutes, the physicians were able to visually see signs of tension and increased movement within the colon itself which subsided only when the student was told the truth—that he did not have any signs of cancer and that it all had been part of the experiment.

Obviously, today's requirement of receiving informed consent from medical volunteers would probably prohibit such a hoax in the name of research. Nevertheless, the experiment was important—especially to those of us who struggle to cope with the symptoms of IBS—in that it showed most visibly the effects of emotion on the colon.

But most IBS sufferers don't need researchers to tell them that stress aggravates their condition. We know it firsthand, after many years of painful awareness.

"I've had problems with my stomach since childhood," a thirty-three-year-old travel agent said as she puffed away on a cigarette. "From the time I was about nine until I reached my teen years, I'd get nauseated whenever I got excited. Just thinking about going to a movie could cause me to throw up.

"Although I've outgrown that pattern, emotions and what they do to me still plague my digestive tract. For me, tension equals pain and constipation. I don't know how to walk slowly. I work ten hours a day and love it. I'm the original Miss Hyper." She smiled wryly. "And I pay for it. My husband calls me 'Miss Rocket Ass.' I *know* stress is making me hurt, but I can't seem to change. I can handle things when my staff makes mistakes; what I can't cope with is when *I* make mistakes. I'm supposed to be perfect."

Stress and the amount of wear and tear it inflicts on the physical body varies according to each person. Each person's "breaking point" differs, and it may even vary for that one person, depending on what else is going on in his or her life. Thus, you might work well under tension and actually feel that you're "addicted to adrenaline," as one woman told me. But when her underage son was arrested for driving while drinking and the next day her mother had a stroke, she was overstressed. Her IBS symptoms returned and she found herself in physical agony.

Another woman told of "too much of a good thing." She got engaged, received a promotion that required her moving to another locale, and won a trip for two to Hawaii. "Everything was positive, really great," she said. "I should have been happy. Yet each success brought problems I'd have to work out. I felt overwhelmed. My irritable bowel syndrome was as bad as it has ever been and I should have been feeling great! Instead, I felt lousy."

Stress is like rainfall: A little may not be harmful. Indeed, it may be good. But too many drops soon erode even the hardest granite. Stress—even "good" stress—piling up too long and too fast can wear down the sturdiest among us.

In 1967, Drs. Thomas H. Holmes and Richard H. Rahe, psychiatrists at the University of Washington Medical School, devised a scale of stressful events which they called

"The Social Readjustment Rating Scale." Some of the life events were "good," such as getting married or outstanding personal achievement. Others were "bad," such as death of a spouse or being fired. Their findings revealed that change—good or bad—created stress which makes an individual more vulnerable to illness.

The following chart, developed by Drs. Thomas H. Holmes and Richard H. Rahe, gives points to various life changes. Check off those which apply to you and total your score.

THE SOCIAL READJUSTMENT RATING SCALE[7]

Rank	Event	Value	You
1	Death of a spouse	100	
2	Divorce	73	
3	Marital separation	65	
4	Jail term	63	
5	Death of a close family member	63	
6	Personal injury/severe illness	53	
7	Marriage	50	
8	Fired at work	47	
9	Marital reconciliation	45	
10	Retirement	45	
11	Change in health of close family member	44	
12	Pregnancy	40	
13	Sex difficulties	39	
14	Gain of a new family member	39	
15	Business readjustment	39	
16	Change in financial state	38	
17	Death of a close friend	37	
18	Change to different work or school major	36	
19	Change in number of arguments w/spouse	35	
20	Home mortgage over $30,000	31	
21	Loan foreclosure/stress of unpaid bills	30	
22	Change in work/school responsibilities	29	
23	Son/daughter leaving home	29	

24	Trouble with in-laws	29
25	Outstanding personal achievement	28
26	Spouse begins or stops work	26
27	Begin or end school	26
28	Revision of personal habits	24
29	Trouble with boss or school instructors	23
30	Change in work or social hours	20
31	Change in residence	20
32	Change in schools	20
33	Change in recreation	19
34	Change in church activities	18
35	Change in school activities	18
36	Mortgage or loan less than $30,000	17
37	Change in sleeping habits	16
38	Change in number of family get-togethers	15
39	Change in eating habits	15
40	Vacation	13
41	Christmas	12
42	Minor violations of the law	11 ____

Total:

(Note: This scale applies to events you experienced within the past year.)

Scoring
150-199 Mild chance in incurring some form of illness in the next year
200-299 Moderate risk of incurring some form of illness in the next year.
300+   Very likely to suffer serious physical or emotional illness.

In later chapters, when you begin to use the "detection diaries" (see Illustration C) to help track what triggers IBS in you, you'll begin to note specific personal patterns and be able to isolate the combination of emotional, dietary, and stress factors that create problems for you.

In general, however, there are certain types of situations that tend to trigger IBS symptoms in most people with this disorder. They include:

- Fatigue mixed with an "X" factor, which could be almost any food, milk product, or alcohol
- Fatigue combined with stress
- Fatigue in association with travel
- Stress created by anxiety, time pressures, more pollution, etc.
- Stress mixed with almost any food or drink

While no specific stress event seems to trigger IBS in all patients, marital problems, financial concerns, job tensions, and family difficulties seem to rank high. According to many studies, numerous "IBS patients report a relationship between subjective tension or stress and an increase in symptoms. Half of IBS patients also say they can recall an acute episode of psychological distress immediately preceding the first onset of their symptoms."[8]

"I can tell you exactly when I started having problems," an airline executive said. "My husband and I separated, then got a divorce. Six months later, my father had heart by-pass surgery. That year I think I lived in the bathroom. If I wasn't having cramps from diarrhea, I was in pain from constipation and gas. My doctor called it 'a case of nerves'!"

Good foods/Bad foods

Although food, by itself, doesn't cause IBS, it can trigger the symptoms. The majority of physicians interviewed reported that approximately 25 percent of their IBS patients complained that eating made their stomach pain worse. In many patients, eating—especially breakfast—triggers almost immediate diarrhea.

Remember that what you eat does not *cause* irritable bowel syndrome. A particular food, type of food, or combination of foods, however, can trigger symptoms at a specific time in certain individuals.

That means that everyone reacts differently to a particular food. Of course, some people have true allergies to foods or enzyme deficiencies—such as an intolerance to milk products, known as "lactose intolerance." These people usually develop IBS-type symptoms when they eat or drink milk products.

Many people with IBS, on the other hand, develop symptoms only at certain times when they drink milk or eat ice cream. With them, the specific food triggers symptoms only when other internal or external stimuli are present—if they're overly tired, under more stress than usual, or anxious about something.

For many sufferers, just the stress caused by having IBS triggers unpleasant symptoms. It's understandable to have concerns. IBS is a recurring chronic disorder that brings with it pain and discomfort. It may go away for weeks, months, or even years and you think you're cured—only to have the symptoms pop back up like a witch in an amusement park's haunted house. No wonder you may feel frustrated, depressed, angry, and worried.

It's natural. Your body's acting up—a very personal and private part of your body—and no one seems to know why or be able to cure you. You wonder if you're really all right or if, perhaps, there's actually something seriously wrong and no one's telling you—or worse, the doctors have misdiagnosed it.

You're not alone in these feelings. It's hard not to have doubts when you've been x-rayed and had barium enemas, sigmoidoscopy, stool cultures, and other tests and everything's coming up negative. You may be relieved but at the same time worried. If you're like most people with IBS, you've had a number of physical problems over the years, such as appendicitis, gallbladder problems, menstrual difficulties if you're female, and vague stomach or intestinal pains. Studies by Drs. Whitehead and Schuster reveal that patients with IBS tend to be more preoccupied with illness than subjects without IBS. Could it be because they feel only "fair to middling" much of the time?

See your physician

That's why it's so important for you to get proper medical advice. Once your doctor has examined you and run tests, ruling out serious disease and giving you the diagnosis of "irritable bowel syndrome," you need to be sure you feel comfortable with your doctor/patient relationship. You must be able to discuss your fears and concerns with your physician.

Don't increase stress unnecessarily by keeping your worries to yourself. A doctor's goal is to try to make you feel better, both physically and psychologically. Never think your questions are "silly." If you're bothered by something, it's important to get some answers. We often think the doctor should know what's bothering us, but most of them aren't blessed with ESP. The doctor can't read your mind. If you don't ask questions, he or she probably will assume you understand.

Write down your questions in advance so you don't forget them once you're face-to-face with your doctor. You might want to take notes, as well. If you don't understand the answer, say so. Sometimes it's difficult for a physician to translate medical jargon into plain old-fashioned English that a nonmedical person can understand. Your doctor will appreciate your honesty in saying that you need a simpler explanation. Chapter 21 lists many of the questions IBS sufferers ask, along with specific answers. You might want to refer to that chapter if you forget between visits what your doctor told you.

Be sure to be honest in your answers to your doctor, too. Don't be embarrassed. A frank discussion of bowels, diarrhea, or constipation is not going to shock or embarrass your physician. It may be difficult for you at first, as most of us have been trained since childhood to refrain from discussing "bathroom" problems with others, but your doctor must have the necessary background information in order to help you. Saying that you suffer from "constipation," for example, doesn't mean anything to the doctor until you explain what *you* mean by constipation. Does it mean difficulty in moving your bowels? Not having a bowel movement each day? Not having one for a week? Having hard stools?

Be honest and admit it if you use laxatives or take enemas. Overuse of laxatives, often called "laxative-abuse," can cause bowel problems. By sharing that information, you'll save both you and the physician a great deal of time and yourself a number of physical tests and their resulting discomfort and costs.

Also tell your doctor if you're suffering from other problems in your life—marital problems, business concerns, grief from a recent loss of family member or friend. It's typical to feel depressed around the anniversary of someone's death, so be aware of that influence, too, when you're talking to the doctor.

Explain when your symptoms began and what *you* think might have triggered them. When the physician takes your medical history, he or she needs to know more than just the physical pains or discomforts you are experiencing. Illnesses often are a mixture of biological, psychological, and sociocultural factors. Doctors must practice "integrative medicine" and put all these influences together in order to help you. Although IBS patients typically deny or minimize emotional concerns,[9] they do experience them and, as with everyone else, are affected by them to some degree.

Because IBS is a chronic disorder—like diabetes—it cannot be cured. But by communicating openly and honestly with your physician—saying what is or isn't effective and describing when and under what circumstances you have symptoms and how you feel—you can develop the understanding necessary to take a more active role in managing your irritable bowel syndrome. In the long run, you're the one who has to be responsible for yourself. The doctor is there to treat and advise you, but no physician can be by your side twenty-four hours a day. It is your illness, not your doctor's.

In the "Treatment" section of this book, you'll learn how to begin to change or control those situations you have identified as being stressful for you and how to best reduce the stress itself.

The pain you feel is very real. There is no magical treatment to cure you or to erase the discomfort you experience all too frequently. But by understanding what triggers IBS in you, you can learn to control some of the factors triggering your symptoms and gain relief from IBS.

Dietary Considerations

Eating may be hazardous to your health

"I don't seem to have any IBS problems," an artist confided, "until I eat! Then all hell breaks loose."

She's not alone in her experience. But food, in and of itself, does not cause irritable bowel syndrome. That's important to remember because most of your friends and family will probably dismiss or at least rationalize your symptoms by saying, "It's probably something you ate."

But food doesn't cause irritable bowel syndrome. It's eating it that can be a trigger for IBS symptoms. The actual act of eating triggers movement in the colon, called gastrocolic reflex, in everyone. That's why mothers trying to toilet train their children put them on the potty right after mealtime, especially breakfast. That's when most people have a bowel movement.

But with IBS patients, eating—especially eating a large meal—can trigger more than a leisurely trip to the bathroom. It can set off a tremendous sense of urgency and chronic diarrhea.

According to Dr. Marvin M. Schuster, researchers have learned that in IBS patients, food—just the actual act of eating—can set off extreme hypermotility in the colon within fifty minutes or after beginning the meal. In those without IBS, the motor response induced by eating normally quiets down within fifty minutes. But in IBS sufferers

44

the response not only continues after eating, but also gradually gets stronger. There are ways—both medical and non-medical—to deal with this overresponse. They will be described fully in the section called, "Treating."

Lactose intolerance

Although studies thus far have shown no specific food intolerance unique to IBS patients, about 20 to 40 percent of patients with IBS also have a lactose intolerance. This is the inability to digest lactose, the main sugar found in milk and other dairy products. The result is stomach bloating, cramplike abdominal pain, gas, and diarrhea—which also are symptoms of irritable bowel syndrome. In fact, the symptoms are indistinguishable.

In addition, approximately 30 percent of those people who see a physician with symptoms of irritable bowel syndrome discover they actually have a lactose intolerance. As approximately 25% of the American adult population suffers from this inability to digest milk and milk products, it's quite possible that you may be one of them. Your physician can determine whether or not you have a lactose intolerance by either putting you on a two- or three-week lactose-free diet or by administering a lactose intolerance test. Until you find out for sure if your symptoms are caused by lactose intolerance, you might want to eliminate milk and other dairy products from your diet to see if your symptoms lessen.

Remember that cheese and butter, even if they're blended with other foods, are still milk products, so if you choose to try a lactose elimination diet you must omit these as well. Dairy products also may hide in bread, cookies and cakes, and many ready-to-eat foods. Check the labels.

People react differently to a particular food

Sorry, you'll get no list of "foods to avoid." They truly differ from person to person. One woman reported that "green or red peppers act like poison to me. They're worst when they're cooked because then they affect everything else in the dish. Within an hour of eating them I get diarrhea, cramps, and nausea.'' Many other IBS sufferers, however, eat peppers—red or green—with no symptoms whatsoever.

What's more, a specific food may trigger symptoms of IBS in an individual only when other internal or external stimuli are also present, such as fatigue or stress.

That's why I usually can enjoy cooked cabbage chased down with hot coffee while my friend with IBS studiously avoids both, as cabbage (like beans) produces increased intestinal gas and coffee (as well as cola drinks and chocolate) stimulates bowel action. But when I'm under stress or overly fatigued, I also abstain from cabbage and coffee because both affect me adversely at those times. My friend eliminates red wine and artichokes when she's under stress because then, and only then, these foods cause an almost immediate pain, gas, and frequent diarrhea.

Some IBS sufferers, however, abstain from foods they think trigger problems for them, foods that trigger IBS in friends, and even foods they've read are ''bad'' for people with stomach and intestinal problems of any type. They remember a parent or grandparent who had stomach trouble and was treated with a soft, bland diet (the pre-1970s treatment for people with irritable bowel syndrome and other similar disorders),[1] and emulate that person. Before too long, they end up with an unbalanced diet that aggravates their IBS symptoms rather than alleviating them.

''The problem with eliminating foods from your diet too quickly,'' says Dr. Douglas A. Drossman, ''is that if you become too zealous, you can soon find yourself with little or nothing to eat. I've had a few patients who cut out everything but baby food because they were sure everything else triggered their IBS.''

On the other hand, there are some foods, such as wheat, corn, citrus fruits, and tea, which are known to trigger symptoms in many IBS patients. They may not present a problem to you, however. For those for whom they are a problem, there is an irony, as wheat bran often is prescribed to add fiber to one's diet. Determining which foods, if any, are problems and under what situations is a highly individualized problem and is what makes your detection diaries (which you'll learn about in the "Tracking" section) all the more important.

While doctors tend to disagree over the number of IBS patients who actually have true food intolerances, a 1985 British study involving 122 patients identified a large number of foods producing symptoms in these IBS sufferers.[2] Only 5 percent of the patients tested had intolerances to one food alone while 32 percent had intolerances to eleven or more of the foods.

Food	% of patients intolerant
Cereals	
Wheat	60
Corn	44
Oats	34
Rye	30
Barley	24
Rice	15
Dairy Products	
Milk	44
Cheese	39
Butter	25
Yogurt	24
Fish	
White fish	10
Shell fish	10
Smoked fish	7
Meat	
Beef	16
Pork	14
Chicken	13
Lamb	11
Turkey	8
Fruit	
Citrus	24

Food	% of patients intolerant
Apples	12
Rhubarb	12
Bananas	11
Strawberries	8
Pineapple	8
Pears	8
Grapes	7
Melon	5
Avocado pear	5
Raspberries	4

Vegetables

Onions	22
Potatoes	20
Cabbage	19
Sprouts	18
Peas	17
Carrots	15
Lettuce	15
Leeks	15
Broccoli	14
Soybeans	13
Spinach	13
Mushrooms	12
Parsnips	12
Tomatoes	11
Cauliflower	11
Celery	11
Green beans	10
Cucumber	10
Turnips	10
Beetroot	8
Peppers	6

Miscellaneous

Coffee	33
Eggs	26
Tea	25
Chocolate	22
Nuts	22
Preservatives	20

Food	% of patients intolerant
Yeast	12
Sugar beet	12
Sugarcane	12
Alcohol	12
Tap water	10
Saccharin	9
Honey	2

While this study lists many of the items that other researchers, as well as patients, have found to be triggers for IBS symptoms, remember that the sampling was small, involving only 122 patients. Do *not* assume that every food on this list can cause problems for you. Don't let food become a scapegoat when you're trying to track down what triggers IBS.

Some foods do create gas in many people, including those without IBS. Onions, beans, brussels sprouts, and cabbage are some of the most common offenders, but again, this does not mean that they are bad for you. Sorbitol-containing gum also can trigger gas and diarrhea in some people, especially those who chew with their mouths open or who blow bubbles, as both practices cause you to swallow excessive air. Xanthine-containing beverages may trigger excessive diarrhea in some IBS sufferers.

Fat and fiction

Fat—in the form of animal fat, oil, or butter—does stimulate colonic contractions in most people. Therefore, it should be no surprise to learn that some IBS patients, especially those who have had their gallbladders removed, find that fatty foods, such as pork, bacon, and fried foods especially, consistently seem to trigger their symptoms, usually gas, diarrhea, and stomach pains. The symptoms may be caused by the hormone cholecystokinin (also known as CCK), which is released when we eat to help the small intestine digest food, especially fatty foods. If you find your symptoms returning or increasing after eating fried foods or those containing a great deal of fat or grease, it's probably a good idea to reduce your intake or eliminate them from your meals.

Fiber: fact and fantasy

Even though fiber—ingested through foods, bran, or bulking agents (such as Metamucil or Konsyl)—is important in treating IBS (you'll read a great deal about how to include more of it in your diet in the section on ''Treating''), some people react badly to extra fiber. Some, as mentioned before, can't tolerate wheat. Others find that their digestive tract becomes more severely irritated when they eat fiber-rich food. Many physicians recommend using commercial psyllium seed preparations rather than eating additional bran, but you need to check with your physician to see what he or she determines is best for you.

Most people experience some additional gas at first when they add extra fiber to their diet, much of which dissipates in four to six weeks, when the intestine gets used to the extra bulk. Only a small percentage of people react with such violent gas pains and severe diarrhea that additional fiber is not a good idea for them. This just underlines the importance of understanding your individual body system and how it reacts to various stimuli when you're trying to uncover what triggers your IBS. Don't give up on the idea of extra fiber too soon. But if you continue to have problems tolerating the higher levels of fiber in your diet, consult your physician.

Childhood food myths

A group of us were sitting over coffee after a lovely dinner in a fashionable restaurant. ''The desserts here are sensational,'' said one man, ''but I'd give anything for my mother's egg custard. She used to fix it for me whenever I didn't feel well.''

I have pleasant childhood memories of egg custard, too. My father's department store stayed open on Monday nights, the same night the local Y had its ''teen'' dances for the junior high crowd. My father and I had a regular Monday night dinner date at the Y cafeteria. I ignored the luscious-looking pies and opted instead for the egg custard, served in dark brown ceramic cups and topped with caramelized brown sugar. The memory—of both the egg custard and those dinners alone with my father—was very soothing.

We began to speak of other comfort foods, treats such as ice cream, rice puddings, tapioca, and bread pudding. The English call them "nursery foods," probably because they were served to the children in the nursery by their nannies or because they were among the first solid foods a baby ate. These foods are simple, soft, easy to eat, and somewhat tasteless by adult standards. Yet we hold their memories fondly, in the same section of the brain's scrapbook as hot chocolate topped with whipped cream or marshmallows and, of course, toasted marshmallows burned to a crisp and delicious beyond belief.

A glass of warm milk may have soothed you to sleep at one point in your life, but now it can be your worst enemy. A friend of mine still has not recovered from the night his companionable cup of hot cocoa became his monstrous foe.

Yet our mouths watered as we described these comfort foods. It had been years since any of us had tasted them. But why? We asked the question aloud. All six of us at the table had given up these fondest foods of our childhood because they no longer agreed with us. These "comfort foods" now gave us stomach cramps, gas, and diarrhea. They also contained milk, eggs, and sugar, ingredients that trigger IBS symptoms in many people as well as problems for those with lactose intolerance.

Like mother, like daughter

While dictating a recipe to my teenage daughter, I said, "It calls for nutmeg, but I never use it."

"Why not?" she asked.

I had to stop a minute to consider the question. I not only had never *used* nutmeg, I had never even *tasted* it! Why not? Because my mother never used it.

By the same token, many of us have food likes and dislikes we learned at our parents' table. "Pork's too greasy. I can't digest it." "Onions make me gassy." "I never eat vegetables." Just as I assumed I wouldn't like nutmeg because my mother hadn't, many people ban certain foods from their diet based on their parents' taste. What's more, they may be preconditioned not only to dislike a particular food, but also to react badly to it because they grew up seeing those they loved reacting that way.

The emotional component of food

You won't find "emotion" listed along with sodium content or calorie count on any food product, but it's there and it's a powerful ingredient. There's little doubt that food *can* make us feel ill and can trigger IBS symptoms even if we don't actually eat it.

When I was eight or nine, my sister loved beets. She pleaded with my mother to serve them every night and, on those evenings when they were served, my sister often had two or three helpings. One night she ate more than that. A lot more. Understandably, she was sick to her stomach. Although I was indifferent to beets before then—I ate what was put on my plate but never asked for more—since that day I have never eaten beets. The look and the smell (although I'm not sure they have any scent) make me feel queasy.

Bananas also trigger emotions for me that find their outlet in very physical ways. When I was a child, during the last of the "real" wars—World War II—I developed a serious case of diarrhea (early IBS?) that lasted for weeks. Unable to get bananas because of the wartime food shortages, my mother purchased banana powder that could be reconstituted by adding water. Although I have no real memory of the experience, I still have a strong aversion to bananas and actually become nauseated, gag, and develop stomach pains at the slightest smell of bananas. When my kids were babies, they gobbled down applesauce, strained apricots, and strained peaches, but I never could get my hand to move toward the jars of pureed bananas in the grocery store.

Most people don't have such strong aversions to food. If you do, however, trying to wish it away by calling it "silly" or "just in my head" probably won't fool your digestive system. Emotions are powerful and hold great control over our entire physical being. As one physician said, "Those medical anatomy textbooks are wrong. They really should show the brain attached to the gut."

Foods do *not* cause irritable bowel syndrome. As they often do trigger symptoms, however, you need to discover and eliminate those that present problems for you. In the "Tracking" section of this book, you'll learn how to identify which foods are poor choices for you—for whatever reasons—and in what situations. While omitting these offending foods from your diet won't cure you, it should bring some relief.

6

Other Triggering Considerations

While emotional stress and diet are usually the first two triggering culprits blamed when one has a problem with irritable bowel syndrome, there are other factors that need to be considered before you begin to play detective.

Drugs: prescription, over-the-counter, and illegal

Despite the fact that they are ingested, oral medicines often are not mentioned when someone—doctor or patient—is trying to determine what has triggered unpleasant IBS symptoms. The doctor may not consider medications because the patient neglects to mention what he or she is taking (either prescribed by other physicians or over-the-counter). If the patient does mention some of the medications, he or she often forgets to add specific over-the-counter preparations that are so common we tend to forget they're drugs, too—items such as aspirin, antihistamines, antacids, and iron pills. Yet these preparations often trigger or intensify the symptoms of IBS.

• Laxatives

Laxative overuse is a major trigger of IBS symptoms and is one that is difficult for physicians to determine as many people underestimate their usage of laxatives or deny taking them altogether. Research studies suggest that approximately 24 million Americans use laxatives one to three times a month and 10.6 million use them one or more times a week. Some patients use laxatives so frequently that they take them for granted as part of a routine, like brushing your teeth before going to bed or washing your face in the morning. No wonder these patients fail to mention their laxative use to their physician.

Yet diarrhea is often triggered by the overuse of laxatives. What's more, the more you depend on laxatives to regulate your bowels, the more you'll need to "get the job done." The dosage often has to be increased, then upped again, until soon you may be using far more than the specific dosage recommended by the manufacturer.

Laxatives also may cause other unpleasant side effects, including severe cramps, burning, skin rashes, and upset of normal body chemistry. Those who use laxatives as a form of weight control—most often women who suffer from anorexia and/or bulimia or teenage boys who engage in boxing, wrestling, or other sports with weight requirements—can become addicted to these drugs and find it almost impossible to break the laxative habit.

Long-term users may develop "cathartic colon," a condition in which nerve cells in the colon are damaged and the colon loses its normal shape and responds only to artificial stimuli. This leads to bloating and constipation, both of which are also symptoms of IBS. Fortunately, once the use of laxatives is curtailed, the bowel can be retrained to resume its normal function.

As you can see, laxatives often make worse the very condition they're supposed to overcome! According to Dr. Marvin M. Schuster, "Lifelong laxative abuse may result in laxative dependence with continuing and worsening constipation as a result of increasing tolerance to the laxative."

If you don't take them, don't start. If you do take them, try tapering off and substituting additional natural fiber in your diet instead.

• Antibiotics

Antibiotics, those miracle drugs used and often overused for bacterial and viral infections, also may trigger more problems than they cure. They not only kill off invading germs, they also may destroy the "friendly" organisms that live in our intestines. That can cause diarrhea, a problem whether or not you have IBS as well. With IBS sufferers, however, the diarrhea may continue long after the antibiotic treatment is completed.

In an English study, many women reported having IBS symptoms for the first time following abdominal or pelvic surgery or after receiving antibiotic therapy for one reason or another.[1]

• High blood pressure medications

Drugs that are effective in the treatment of hypertension, such as Inderal, unfortunately can also affect the motility of the colon, which in IBS patients is already abnormal. This can trigger additional diarrhea. It does not mean, however, that you should stop taking your hypertension medication, but rather that you should inform your physician so he or she can try substituting other drugs that will be effective for high blood pressure without making your IBS symptoms worse.

• Nicotine

Nicotine, taken into the body through smoking, can irritate the colon. It also may exacerbate IBS symptoms as it is a laxative. For this and other well-documented reasons you already know about, you should do everything in your power to stop smoking. Many hospitals and clinics offer special seminars to help smokers wean themselves from this most self-destructive habit. Check your newspaper or contact your local hospitals, American Red Cross, or American Cancer Society.

• Narcotics

Other drugs can upset your bowels, too. Narcotics, such as heroin, codeine, and morphine, can cause constipation. If you see someone other than your regular physician when you have a cough or cold, be sure that the doctor also knows you have irritable bowel syndrome. Otherwise you may get a prescription for a cough medicine containing codeine.

• Diuretics

Diuretics, often known as water pills, also can trigger constipation because they draw fluid out of the stools. Never "borrow" someone else's water pills to help you lose weight. As a matter of fact, you should never use anyone else's prescription drug.

• Alcohol

Although many people tend to forget that alcohol is a drug, it is and can cause diarrhea in some people. Wine, in particular, seems to bother many IBS sufferers, although red wine seems to be more often the culprit than white. Beer may create gas and excessive bloating in some people.

Hormones

The body's own drug system—the hormonal system—often triggers IBS symptoms in those susceptible. Cholecystokinin (known as CCK), for example, is just one of many hormones released by the body to help with the digestion of fats. CCK not only makes you feel full after you eat a high fat content meal, but it also stimulates the colon so the food can move through the digestive tract faster. Many doctors feel that, in people with IBS, the hormone moves the food along too fast, which is why many irritable bowel sufferers get diarrhea soon after eating a rich meal (e.g., pork chops, duck, cheesecake, etc.).

The hormone progesterone also affects colon motility and can trigger IBS symptoms. Many women report bowel upsets prior to menstruation. "I usually am constipated a few days before my period begins," an accountant said. "Then when my period starts, I have diarrhea for two days. It's been that way for years. I never knew until recently that other women had the same problem. My gynecologist never said anything about it—of course, I never mentioned I had a problem, either!''

What triggers it in me?

That's the question you must begin to ask. The next section, "Tracking," shows you how to go about sorting out and becoming aware of those things in your daily life that work against you, triggering IBS in you.

Remember that irritable bowel syndrome is a chronic disease. You're not going to get over it. But when you know what triggers it, you can then begin to reduce some of the symptoms and learn how to cope with the others.

═══ TRACKING ═══

TRACKING

7

Tools For Tracking

What now?

The easy part is over! No one really knows what actually causes IBS, what triggers it, or what to do about it, and the most difficult task is trying to zero in on what triggers it in you. Since each person differs, the typical "things to avoid" checklist handed out by your physician when you're trying to lose weight or lower high blood pressure doesn't work. You need a highly personalized list, one that it's up to you to determine, if you're going to successfully track down what triggers IBS symptoms in you.

Don't expect it to be a simple search. The human memory is selective. Just as we get accustomed to the clutter around us, we tend to take for granted those things—experiences, emotions, food, tension—that might be triggering our IBS.

Before you begin to reorganize a room and strip it of unnecessary clutter, you need to first take a photograph of it. Those things you tend to ignore or look right through when you see them on a daily basis become very obvious in a snapshot. A kitchen countertop covered with magazine clippings, an overdue library book, one soccer shin guard, a bottle of sunscreen, a screwdriver, and a malfunctioning calculator suddenly become quite visible in a picture.

By the same token, when you're trying to track down what triggers IBS symptoms, you need to record each day's events and activities as accurately as you can. It's harder than taking a photo, of course, because you have to chronicle not only what you eat, for example, but also when, what's happening to you and around you, and what emotional setting you're in or experiencing from past memories. Your colon isn't isolated; it's part of you, and whatever involves you in any way also can affect your colon.

Be patient! Recording this data is not an exact science. You're not going to get the answers immediately. It's not like getting on a scale and discovering right away that you've lost two pounds or having your blood pressure taken and getting an instantaneous reading. You won't get a computer printout of numbers that can then be translated into a tidy list of dos and don'ts. That makes it tough, because most of us are used to "one-minute solutions."

Sorry. You're going to have to find your answers slowly and by trial and error. You may think that you've found something that is "bad" for you and swear never to eat or drink it again, only to find that the next time you do, your digestive tract behaves beautifully and you have no unpleasant reaction. On the other hand, you may regularly eat something like dill pickles or popcorn and suffer no reaction whatsoever, only to find that when you're under a great deal of stress these foods cause you to double up with pain and diarrhea.

As no one's quite figured out just how to take snapshots of emotion, fatigue, or stress, you'll have to try the next best thing. Consider using the "detection diary" (Illustration C) to jog your memory and help you to play Sherlock Holmes as you track down what triggers IBS in you.

How to use the detection diaries

Although there are many ways to record your mood, diet, fatigue level, and other variables, I find the detection diaries to be the handiest and most efficient because they fit in your pocket or purse, are quick and simple to fill out, and can be arranged in various ways to help show you—visually— what bothers you and under what circumstances.

Keeping food diaries in a notebook often becomes tedious and after a week or two most of us play "catch up"—wondering, was it Wednesday or Thursday that we had the pizza and did we have a drink before dinner?—and trying to fill in all the blanks before returning to the doctor. No wonder so many physicians question the validity of our diaries!

Food diaries by themselves also often omit the emotional and fatigue components of your meals, factors that usually are inseparable when trying to track down triggering causes for IBS. They also ignore medications you may be taking, your past experiences, your stress level, and your learned responses for various behaviors. These and other ingredients play an important role in triggering your IBS symptoms.

The detection diary, on the other hand, combines a number of factors: mood, time of day, food or drink ingredient, symptoms, and what you think was the triggering agent. You can either duplicate the detection diary example (see Illustration C), copy it on index cards, or send $1 (in check or money order made out to Elaine Fantle Shimberg) per preprinted pad, and a stamped, self-addressed #10 envelope, to:

Elaine Fantle Shimberg
IBS
P.O. Box 3369
Tampa, FL 33601-3369

Try to fill out the detection diaries routinely at mealtimes as well as each time you feel any symptoms. Make them as complete as possible, not only recording the time of day but also noting your mood, whether you've eaten (and if so, what), and any other facts that may be pertinent, such as unusual stress you're under and things happening in your life (job change, marital problems, visiting relatives, troubles with kids, financial difficulties). Trust nothing to memory. Write legibly and if you use abbreviations, make sure you remember what they mean. A week later you may not recall whether "FAT" meant "fatigued" or "fatty meal."

While you don't want to become too introspective and examine every aspect of your daily life under a microscope, you should become aware of mood and tension patterns that keep cropping up during or just before you experience pain, diarrhea, gas, or other symptoms. You are the only one who can track this. Your doctor, regardless of how capable, won't be able to ferret them out. He or she will, however, be able to help you look over a few weeks' worth of detection diaries to try to discover patterns or triggering trends.

Remember to also record any prescription medicine you may be taking or any drugs (including alcohol) that could be affecting you. Ophthalmic (eye) medications should also be considered as they are absorbed into your system through the mucous membranes. Be alert for any effects from any over-the-counter drugs, especially those you may take so regularly (such as antacids or laxatives) that you tend to forget about them.

When you list what you've eaten, also record any spices that may have been added, as these can turn a "safe" dish (e.g., spaghetti with butter and parmesan cheese) into a potential trigger (e.g., spaghetti with peppers and a garlic sauce).

Since IBS symptoms tend to wax and wane, you need to accumulate a minimum of two to three weeks' worth of the detection diaries to get a good sampling of the times that you are having problems.

Then spread the cards on a flat surface, such as a table or the floor. Move them around in groupings; try to note similarities. If you begin to see a pattern—such as having more symptoms when you're fatigued and eat a late dinner, or after business meetings when your boss is in attendance, or when you skip breakfast and then eat a heavy lunch— you may have begun to track down some of your triggering situations.

Check locations, too. Do you tend to have more symptoms at home? In the office? At meetings? One woman discovered she began to feel nauseated and experience IBS

ILLUSTRATION C

Trigger: _____   Symptoms: _____

Exercise: _____   Stress factors: _____

Stomach: ☐ empty ☐ with food/drink _____

Mood: ☐ normal ☐ angry ☐ fatigued
       ☐ frustrated ☐ bored ☐ anxious
       ☐ other_____

Time: A.M. 1 2 3 4 5 6 7 8 9 10 11 Noon
      P.M. 1 2 3 4 5 6 7 8 9 10 11 Midnight
Relief from IBS: Elaine Fantle Shimberg

Trigger: _____   Symptoms: _____

Exercise: _____   Stress factors: _____

Stomach: ☐ empty ☐ with food/drink _____

Mood: ☐ normal ☐ angry ☐ fatigued
       ☐ frustrated ☐ bored ☐ anxious
       ☐ other_____

Time: A.M. 1 2 3 4 5 6 7 8 9 10 11 Noon
      P.M. 1 2 3 4 5 6 7 8 9 10 11 Midnight
Relief from IBS: Elaine Fantle Shimberg

ILLUSTRATION D

Trigger: *Caesar salad* Symptoms: *diarrhea*

Exercise: *none* Stress factors: *rushed*

Stomach: ☑ empty ☐ with food/drink _____

Mood: ☑ normal ☐ angry ☐ fatigued
       ☐ frustrated ☐ bored ☐ anxious
       ☐ other_____

Time: A.M. 1 2 3 4 5 6 7 8 9 10 11 (Noon)
      P.M. 1 2 3 4 5 6 7 8 9 10 11 Midnight

Relief from IBS: Elaine Fantle Shimberg

Trigger: *Missed plane* Symptoms: *cramps & diarrhea*

Exercise: *none* Stress factors: *Tension*

Stomach: ☐ empty ☑ with food/drink *1 glass white wine*

Mood: ☐ normal ☑ angry ☑ fatigued
       ☑ frustrated ☐ bored ☐ anxious
       ☐ other_____

Time: A.M. 1 2 3 4 5 6 7 8 9 10 11 Noon
      P.M. 1 2 3 4 5 6 7 8 9 (10) 11 Midnight

Relief from IBS: Elaine Fantle Shimberg

pain as soon as she entered a particular restaurant. When she admitted that it had been the favorite dining spot for her and her ex-husband while they were still married, she realized that the atmosphere of that particular watering hole was still too electric for her to handle.

While some other people find it helpful to trade information with others, you're probably better off discussing your symptoms only with your physician. First of all, it prevents you from subconsciously comparing yourself with someone else. Remember, what may be a minor irritation to your friend could be one of your major triggers.

Also, only your physician is trained to look at the total picture of your symptoms and your body's personal quirks, and then to help you to interpret your detection diaries.

A third reason for sharing your symptoms only with your physician is that friends and family, no matter how loving and loyal, soon tire of hearing "organ recitals." They may request equal time, and goodness knows you really don't want to hear *their* list of symptoms, do you?

Many physicians suggest that you try to focus on the times you're feeling good as much as possible, rather than on trying to analyze each twinge to determine if it might be leading up to major discomfort.

Mood mapping

Most researchers agree that IBS sufferers have increased motility in the colon and/or small intestine. But according to Drs. William E. Whitehead and Marvin M. Schuster, under resting conditions (i.e., when the patients have neither eaten nor had medication and are free from as much emotional stress as possible in a test situation), the IBS patients tend to have more or less the same colon movement as "normal" subjects. When stimulated by drugs, hormones, or stress, however, those with IBS tend to have more colonic movement than those free from the disorder. Obviously, then, emotion is an important factor to consider when tracking down what triggers your IBS.

Psychological tests consistently show IBS patients to score

significantly higher than nonpatients in turning anxiety into physical symptoms and in feeling hostile and depressed.[1]

That doesn't mean IBS is in your head, however. It means that because of the abnormalities in your gut, you turn stress, anxiety, and anger into increased colon motility, whereas another person under stress might experience migraine headaches or increased blood pressure. According to Dr. W. Grant Thompson, "Emotion may trigger an abnormal response from individuals with a physiologically abnormal gut."[2]

Rather than wasting time and energy (and emotion) defending yourself as an emotionally strong man (or woman), arguing over whether or not anxiety hits you in the gut, try accepting that most researchers and practicing physicians and psychologists think that it does. Then do yourself a favor by actively tracking down your emotional triggers.

Identify stressors in your life

Obviously, one person's stressors may not be another's. You can't borrow your best friend's list. Loud music turns my intestines into knots; my best friend not only loves to "feel the vibration" from the music, she also can write better while it's pulsating. I sit in my silent cavelike study and marvel at the uniqueness of people.

You might as well acknowledge that uniqueness, accepting that each of us is different and that our frustration levels differ as well. You also need to be honest with yourself about what bothers you. Sometimes we don't want to admit that people—especially those we love or care for—might be a source of stress. But sometimes they are. It's even possible that, on rare occasions, *we* trigger stress in others as well.

• People

Sometimes people create anger in us, an emotion that so worries or embarrasses us that we keep it inside, where it triggers symptoms of IBS rather than expressing it either verbally or in some other physical way, such as developing a migraine or a stiff neck.

"I'm a people person," a forty-year-old insurance salesman said. "I wouldn't be much good in this job if I weren't." Then he hesitated a minute. "I *like* people, but sometimes they really get to me. I'll spend hours with someone, listening to his needs and really trying to put together a good insurance package for him. Then, after I make this really great proposal, he'll say, 'Thanks, but I've got a nephew who really takes care of all my insurance.' I can just feel my stomach knot up."

This phenomenon is common enough that it's invaded our language. "He gives me a pain in the gut," "He's really got guts," "I can't stomach him," and "You'll have to 'gut it out,' " are just a few of many similar examples.

Many of us have learned to cope fairly well with strangers and business associates, but those we love really get to us. Thirty-nine-year-old Paula discovered that her mother was a major IBS trigger for her.

"My husband and I usually go to my mother's for Friday night Sabbath dinner. We have for years unless something special comes up. I usually have trouble with pain and diarrhea all weekend. I always thought it was the wine or my mother's chicken soup. When I begged off the soup, she made such a fuss that I ate it to keep her quiet. Then I felt the familiar rumblings and thought, 'Here I go again!'

"Then I began keeping the detection diaries. Was I surprised at the information they gave me. It wasn't the wine or the soup. *Every* time I ate with Mother, no matter where or when or what I ate, my IBS acted up! I started to record how I felt. I discovered I always worried that Mother either would nag about my not eating enough—so I'd order more than I usually ate—or that I'd eat too much and she'd complain about that.

"Finally, I told her that I was almost forty. She couldn't control my eating anymore. I'd either be fat or thin, but it was up to me. That conversation defused a little of my tension when we're together although we both have setbacks every so often."

Occasionally, the people who act as triggers are those we know in social settings. Eight of twenty women IBS sufferers interviewed for this book admitted that they tend to suffer from IBS symptoms while getting ready to attend a social event—a cocktail party, dinner party, concert, or business-related function. Whether it is the situation itself which acts as the trigger or the other people who will be attending is hard to say. The women themselves seemed unable to answer for certain. Each of them said she felt comfortable in the particular setting or, at least, thought she did. None felt threatened by either the situation or others in attendance, but each of these women admitted she experienced serious discomfort from bloating, gas, diarrhea, and abdominal pain. Three of the interviewees said their symptoms had been so bad at times that they were unable to attend a particular function.

To help track down what specifically acts as a trigger before a social situation, you need to use the detection diary to record how you feel about the event itself. Are you resentful about going? Nervous about how you'll look or act? Insecure about not having the proper outfit to wear? Worried about making "small talk"? Did you ever really mess up at a social event, maybe spilling wine on the tablecloth or bumping into a waiter who was carrying a tray of hors d'oeuvres?

Do you nibble before going out? One woman tracked down her pre-social trigger: Before going out to a party she always had a glass of milk to "coat her stomach" before she started drinking alcohol. She discovered that, along with her IBS, she, like 30 percent of others with IBS, also suffered from lactose intolerance. The milk triggered her symptoms. A few pieces of cheese with some crackers would have done the same.

• Places

Particular places can also trigger symptoms, especially when these locations evoke strong emotions. Just going to your office, particularly when you're concerned about job security or are unhappy with your work, can set your colon into abnormal activity. So can returning to school, visiting a hospital, or going to the airport.

Use the detection diaries to record not only what you've eaten, the time of day, and your mood, but also the emotion you feel when visiting a particular place or even thinking about going there. Try to remember any childhood events that may be infiltrating those emotions. Track down even the vaguest of memories. Ask your siblings, parents, other relatives, and friends. Someone may remember the traumatic stay at the hospital as a toddler that you've blocked out of your mind or your embarrassment at forgetting the piano piece at your recital when you were six.

You may track down other places as triggers for your symptoms, too. A noisy bar plus the stress of wondering if you'll meet anyone plus the drug, alcohol, can turn cocktail hour into nightmare time. Is it the tension from the sound level of the music? Stress? Alcohol? Yes, it could be a combination of any or all of these.

Twenty-six-year-old Sandi is a time management specialist. She travels all over the country giving seminars and lectures on her favorite subject. "I love to travel; I love my subject; I love to give speeches," she said. "Why do I have such terrible pain and diarrhea right before I go on?"

When she began keeping detection diaries, she discovered that she really only had symptoms when she presented all-day seminars or evening lectures. When she did morning sessions only, she was fine. What was different? Her diet: She only drank coffee in the afternoon and evening. Caffeine acts as a trigger in many people with IBS and, like nicotine, is a known laxative. In addition, her fatigue level was different. Her morning sessions were after an eight-hour sleep. When she worked all day, she understandably was tired. Her evening lectures were given on top of working a full eight hours.

Sandi eliminated coffee totally, along with other products containing caffeine, such as cola drinks and chocolate, and began taking time off on those days that she also had an evening session. In addition, she shortened her full-day seminars so she could include an hour's catnap for herself. To her amazement, her symptoms let up almost entirely, and when present caused much less discomfort than they had previously.

• Past

This stressor is much more difficult to track down because most of us have selective memory when it comes to our past. We either remember things as far worse than they really were—or much better. One woman recalled her childhood dinner table with great fondness.

"We all sat around the big dinner table," she said, "discussing all kinds of things. It was fascinating."

Her younger sibling, three years her junior, was amazed at the revelation. "*I* sat around that table too," she said. "It wasn't fascinating at all. My father dominated the conversation and we all were supposed to listen in rapt attention. We couldn't talk unless it was something of 'general interest.' How many things of general interest does a nine-year-old have to offer?" Strangely enough, the older sister had no memory of where individual family members sat around that table, while the younger sister remembered not only the exact placement, but also what shape napkin ring everyone had.

Many people with IBS recall the family dinner hour as a time of childhood torment and tension, where misdeeds were examined and exposed to all, punishment doled out, and emotion served up with overcooked gray-looking vegetables.

"I hated our dining table," one IBS sufferer admitted at the intermission of A. R. Gurney, Jr.'s *The Dining Room*, a play centering on the interaction of various families around the traditional dinner table. "My gut was always in agony," he said. "I was so anxious that I couldn't eat and, of course, the more I played with my food, the more hell I got. Even if my parents didn't yell at me and my sisters, I was always afraid that they might. I don't know which was worse, the actual yelling or my fear that something would set them off."

According to Dr. Douglas A. Drossman, that is one of the reasons it's hard to track down what triggers IBS symptoms. Much of the research has been done in hospital and laboratory environments, which are devoid of the emotions of our daily lives. "Furthermore," he states, "the effects of a *symbolic* stimulus (a fantasy or fear) are hard to quantify and may produce profound physiologic effects owing to early experiences or cultural attitudes (e.g., hex, phobias).[3]

• Personality

Is there a typical "IBS personality"? Without exception, each physician and psychologist interviewed for this book said no. Yet there is documentation suggesting that those with IBS often received more attention when ill as children and tend to be more illness-oriented than nonsufferers. How much is more? When is "more" too much? That's difficult to say.

Each person reacts differently to illness, based on many factors including parental role models from childhood, personality, peer expectations, and societal acceptance. The reaction also may vary according to the particular situation. Thus a teenage boy who gets parental attention through illness may begin to demonstrate the same behavior on the football team, until he sees that acceptance by his peers is based on "toughing it out." He quickly becomes "macho" at least with his teammates, and may or may not continue to let his mother fuss over him at home.

A young woman, who typically stayed home from school on the first day of her menstrual cycle, may drag herself to work when she knows her paid sick days are limited. But this is not to say that an individual is malingering if he or she reacts to an illness in a more intense way than others might do. It seldom is a conscious response. Rather, it is part of the emotional behavioral baggage that we have accumulated along our way. Most of us aren't even aware of why we behave as we do.

That's why it's important to look beyond the obvious when tracking what triggers IBS symptoms. In many cases, you are looking for things your unconscious has kept well hidden. Yet in order to treat your symptoms and live to the most normal and fullest extent with this chronic disorder, you must whisk away the cobwebs and look into the shadows.

Studies by Dr. Douglas A. Drossman and his associates indicate that although there is no distinct personality profile of IBS sufferers, these patients do tend to report pain in times of stress and yet "tend to deny or minimize emotional concerns."[4] It's difficult for a doctor to try to understand what triggers symptoms and to suggest a proper course of treatment when the patient ignores or minimizes what's going on or has gone on in his or her life.

Do you worry a lot about your health? Why? Did your parents seem overly concerned about their health? About yours? How did they feel about seeking medical help for you or themselves? How did they feel about health care in general?

How do you feel about negative events in your life? Do you minimize them? Deny them? Try to explain them so they appear to be more positive? Do you feel comfortable saying that negative life experiences are upsetting to you? If you don't, why? Were your parents able to admit it when negative things happened to them?

Do family get-togethers bring you pain, not pleasure? Does traveling tend to make you constipated? Give you diarrhea? Do you dislike using "strange bathrooms"? (Many women tend to.) Why? What life experiences cause you to react with your intestine?

None of us exist in a vacuum, nor can we isolate the effects of the world and its pressures on us and on our bodies. The psychological, social, and biological influences on you as an individual are absolutely and unequivocally intertwined. They must be discovered and exposed in order to best treat your irritable bowel syndrome and help you to gain some control of your symptoms. What exactly are the triggers for *you* and what can you do about them?

=== TREATING ===

Making Changes In Your Life-Style

The remaining chapters deal with ways in which you can treat the symptoms of irritable bowel syndrome. Remember, the goal is to help you find relief from your symptoms, not to make them completely disappear. My intent is to help you minimize the discomfort and inconvenience of your symptoms and begin to focus on feeling good most of the time so you can enjoy life to its fullest.

Any time you try to make changes in your life-style, however, you are bound to have both successes and failures, with probably more failures than successes in the beginning. A life-style is built over the years, step by step. Changes must be made the same way, slowly, deliberately, and persistently.

You may find it difficult to even recognize what needs changing. Most of us have become so addicted to stress that we may not even recognize it, let alone what it does to us physically. Or we may attempt drastic changes without really taking the time to know or understand ourselves.

A busy executive who thrives on pressure, activity, and juggling many business deals seemingly simultaneously and without much effort agreed to take one week off and do nothing at the beach.

"It was the worst week I ever spent," he moaned. "My wife loved the inactivity. She read, knitted, and walked on the beach. *I* was climbing the walls. I felt emotionally drained and physically rotten. My IBS flared up worse than it ever had while I was working.''

One person's leisure is another's agony. That's why it's vital to take the time to understand what gives you pleasure and what creates tension, and to recognize the emotional and physical feelings you have with both.

Don't expect overnight success. The only ''overnight successes'' are a handful of actors and actresses—most of whom have been working hard at becoming an ''overnight success'' for many years.

Also, don't be too hard on yourself when you find you're slipping back into old habits. They're the hardest to break because they've been around so long and, let's face it, good or bad, they're comfortable.

Start small

You have to crawl before you can walk and walk before you can run. Give yourself tiny goals and reward yourself when you succeed. While it's fine to share success stories with others, remember that each person is different and what motivates your friend to change may not influence you at all. It's like dieting. Some people do well in a group environment with peer support, while others prefer to try it alone. Still others give up all control and opt for a passive liquid diet. Discovering the system that works best for you is what's important, not the particular system.

Since IBS symptoms are triggered by stress and emotion, you're obviously going to have to develop ways to reduce stress so it doesn't affect you so greatly. Some of the following chapters describe in detail methods I have used successfully as well as those others have used to cope with stress and emotional situations. Copy them or change and adapt these ideas to suit your personal taste. They're merely a jumping-off place, a guide to help you along the way.

Make a commitment

The beginning of this "changing one's life-style thing" must be to make the commitment. What causes anyone to say, "Today's the day," differs greatly depending on the individual. For a smoker who decided to call it quits, it was realizing how stained her fingers had become. For a previously failed dieter to try once more to lose excess pounds, it was pictures of her taken at a recent family gathering. For me to make specific changes to find relief from IBS, it was a painful attack of cramps and diarrhea and knowing it was triggered because I had let certain people walk all over me once again.

You have to be the one to make the commitment to create certain changes in your life. Your significant other can't do it for you; your best friend can't make you do it; this book won't make you do it. The desire must be yours—because if it is, the success will be yours as well.

Chart your progress

For some reason, most people become more motivated when they can visualize their progress (and failures). While you shouldn't spend so much time designing and painting beautiful charts that you don't have any time left to exercise, it does help you to stay on track when you know you're going to graph your time and mileage when you're finished.

You can also graph the time you've spent practicing relaxation techniques. Actually putting it down in writing tends to formalize the act and also reinforces the suggestion that you need to do it the following day, too.

Be careful, though, that you don't get so carried away with your charts and graphs that you build up new and additional stress by being overly competitive. If you tend to be something of a perfectionist or addictive in your work or eating habits, you'll have to guard against transferring those traits into the very activities that are supposed to relax you.

Rather than making a chart, you might try putting five pennies on your kitchen window ledge or desk top each morning, and moving one to the left each time you take a few minutes out of your day to pause and relax for a few minutes. Or put a quarter in a jar or box to "buy" yourself a five-minute relaxation break. You'll soon have a jar filled with quarters that you can use to buy yourself a special relaxation gift.

Keep a journal. If you're not much for writing, just divide the page in half. On one side, write "What I Did For Me" and on the other half, "How I Felt About It." Many of us scurry about doing what we feel has to be done and what we feel we have to do for others and then discover there's no time left over to make ourselves feel good. When you have IBS, it's extra important to make yourself feel good because when you don't, it hurts.

Think "good" thoughts

You'll hear a lot about positive thinking in the "Treating" section of this book because I agree with Norman Vincent Peale, Norman Cousins, and many others that there is, indeed, power and purpose in thinking that way.

It's easy to feel depressed when you have the pain and discomfort that comes with irritable bowel syndrome. Unfortunately, thinking good thoughts won't cure you of this disorder. But they *can* make you feel better because you'll be focusing on the times you've felt good, rather than on how lousy you feel just now. It isn't being Pollyanna. It's being realistic.

In Norman Cousin's book, *Anatomy of an Illness*, he tells how he, with his doctor's support, was able to mobilize his body's natural healing powers to overcome a serious crippling illness. He tells of his conviction "that the human mind can discipline the body, can set goals for itself, can somehow comprehend its own potentiality and move resolutely forward."[1]

As a youngster you may have felt pain and discomfort, complained, and received special attention from your parents. Possibly that subconsciously reinforced your pains. But childhood is behind you now and you can't change what was. You can, however, change what is.

It's time to break that habit this very day. Each time you find yourself focusing on how badly you feel, stop and visualize feeling good—no, feeling great! Don't put it off another minute. Promise yourself that you'll stop talking about your illness or discussing your symptoms, other than with your doctor at your next appointment. Ask your friends and relatives to cease asking how you feel, even though you know and appreciate that they're concerned about you.

Dr. Marvin M. Schuster suggests that rather than give attention to yourself for feeling bad, you should focus on and reward yourself for feeling healthy. Any time you find yourself thinking about your symptoms, change your thinking and praise yourself for doing so. You *can* change, you know. You have that power. You can only hold one thought in your mind at a time, so if you start thinking about a beautiful spring day, a playful kitten, or whatever brings a smile to *your* face, you can't possibly also be concentrating on your aching gut.

"View your irritable bowel syndrome as you would view a physical disability which you would try to overcome," Dr. Schuster continues. "Rather than give in to the illness, encourage yourself to push yourself to maximal performances as you would if you had visual impairment, hearing deficit, or other physical disability."[2]

Check your priorities

You have to think and keep thinking about your priorities as you make changes in your life-style. Making changes because "the doctor says so" probably won't work, at least not for long. In the first place, you won't have the necessary commitment and motivation, and in the second, because your heart really isn't in it, you may end up with more stress than you had before—and probably more discomfort from your IBS symptoms as well.

You often can alter situational stress—things going on in your life that create too much tension. You can change the situation, avoid it, or reprogram your responses to the situation. None of these choices is easy. Each takes discipline and commitment. The solution may be as major as ending a tension-filled relationship or as minor as driving a longer but more scenic route to work. Sometimes you'll need the help of a member of the clergy or a mental health professional to help you work out your strategies.

If you do seek advice from a member of the clergy, a psychiatrist, a psychologist, or another mental health professional, don't expect *that person* to tell you what to do. It's your life and you must make your own choices. The professional's job is to listen and to help you clarify your thinking. Also, don't expect immediate answers. Discovering what creates stress and anxiety in your life takes time.

If your job is distressing to you and you dread going to work each Monday, perhaps it's time to reevaluate your career path. Do you really need as much money as you're making if the job has actually become painful? A twenty-three-year-old man mentioned this exact situation to me. He was doing well in his job as a researcher and had just received a healthy bonus and a raise as well. His employer was pleased with his work.

"But I really miss mixing with people," he complained. "I'm cooped up in an office all day, writing reports or conducting interviews by phone. I haven't the guts for it." Then he smiled. He really didn't have the guts for it. His colon was complaining about the stress and the resulting gas, bloating, and constipation were hardly subtle clues.

After pondering his situation for three months, the young man came back to me. "I've weighed my possibilities," he said. "I'd rather have a job that paid less if it made me and my gut happier. Life's too short to be this uncomfortable."

He made the change and is happy, although he now is struggling to make ends meet on commission. He's experiencing stress with this, of course, but this time it isn't bothering him. It must have been a good move because his irritable bowel syndrome is dormant for the time being. That's not to say he's cured, of course. IBS is a chronic disorder. But this young man made an important change in his life-style and, for the time being, he's comfortable with his decision. He's also learned an important lesson: not to be passive in life, but to make changes that are needed when they're needed.

You can always learn new tricks

For me, the most important life-style change was when I learned to be assertive and began to practice time management techniques. I took a noncredit course in assertiveness training and attended a few time management seminars at our local university. These classes truly did change my life and were the beginning of my finding relief from IBS. I think these skills are so important that I'm devoting the next chapter on "Developing Coping Skills" to just two specific skills: being assertive and managing your time.

What I learned in the assertiveness training class and from the few time management lectures I attended was probably nothing I didn't already know subconsciously. But I had just never considered these things to be important skills or tools that could change my life. But they *are* most valuable skills and they *have* changed my life.

I not only learned what these skills were, but much more importantly, I learned how to use them—self-consciously at first, but then as second nature. These skills helped put me in control of my life and helped reduce the stress that triggered my painful bouts of IBS. This sense of being in control is vital in learning to reduce stress in your life. I'll happily share these skills with you in the next chapter.

Developing Coping Skills

Few physicians today deny that irritable bowel syndrome is a disease with a physical basis—an abnormal nervous system in the gut. But they also agree that stress can create flare-ups in this sensitive area, triggering painful symptoms of diarrhea, constipation, an alternating combination of the two, gas, and bloating. In recent studies, IBS patients reported more stress preceding illness than other medical patients or healthy subjects.[1]

When Dr. Douglas A. Drossman and his co-workers in North Carolina studied 566 subjects from a nonpatient population, they found that 15 percent of them had bowel dysfunction compatible with the symptoms of IBS.[2] Yet within this group, 60 percent had never been to a doctor for this complaint.

What makes one person seek medical help while another doesn't? The discomfort level of those who didn't see a doctor seemed to be the same as that of those who went. Perhaps it was how they were raised, whether their parents (usually the mother) tended to take them to the doctor when they didn't feel well or whether they adopted a "wait and see" attitude. Most of us tend to copy our parents' behavior when it comes to illness. If Mom and Dad ignored discomfort and minimized pain, we probably will, too. On the other hand, if they practically had standing appointments with the doctor each week and appeared with complaint list in hand, we may tend to subconsciously inventory ourselves upon waking to see what hurts today.

It also has a great deal to do with the culture we live in. In India, for example, where men traditionally seek health care more often than women, the ratio of men to women diagnosed as having IBS is two to one, just the reverse of that in the United States and Britain.[3]

Whether or not we seek out medical care may also have something to do with how we handle stress. Those of us with more difficulty handling stress may feel more pain and be more likely to see a doctor to make us "feel better."

Although the remainder of this book deals with various ways in which we can reduce our stress level and our discomfort from IBS symptoms, this particular chapter deals with just two: becoming assertive and managing time. By becoming more proficient in these two abilities, we can reduce the negative stress in our lives because we will have more control over our lives. We will actively make decisions that affect us rather than passively react to structures and schedules inflicted on us by others. We'll have more self-esteem and begin to take better care of ourselves in other areas as well.

Obviously, there isn't space in one book to go into great detail on both of these important subjects. But this chapter will deal with the general principles of both assertiveness and time management and show how they relate to relieving stress in those people who have irritable bowel syndrome. There will also be a list of suggested reading for those who would like to learn more about both of these valuable skills.

What is assertiveness?

Assertiveness—it's so easy for some and so very difficult for many of us. It basically means standing up for yourself so other people don't inflict their desires on you. It means expressing your feelings verbally and honestly, and taking the responsibility for those feelings. It is accepting your position as an adult, a person who consciously makes decisions affecting him- or herself and who refuses to be manipulated or made to feel guilty by another.

Why is it important?

It's important to learn to become assertive because it makes us feel better when we are and because if we don't determine and express what we want, others may do it for us. That makes us feel put upon, frustrated, and out of control. It creates stress. We may do what others have chosen for us, but we're fighting that same action internally. Our body will never end up the winner in that battle. Interestingly, the majority of the IBS sufferers interviewed for this book admitted to having great difficulty being assertive. They also acknowledged that the stress created by this inability often triggered symptoms from their oversensitive intestinal tract.

How do we learn to be assertive?

We come into this world with a natural talent for being assertive. When an infant is hungry, he or she cries and lets the caretaker know. There's no hesitation or thoughts of, "Well, this may not be a good time for Mom to feed me. She's too busy," or, "Will Dad still love me if I keep him awake by crying all night?"

Yet as we grow older, many of us (unfortunately, it *does* tend to be something of a female trait) tend to suppress our needs, wanting to please and not "create waves." So we don't say it's inconvenient to stop to pick up the laundry or that we'd really rather not run over to feed your cats while you're on vacation. Instead we deny our feelings, smile, and say, "Of course I will," and wonder why those familiar intestinal rumblings are beginning again. We not only don't feel good, we don't feel good about ourselves and we turn that anger inside.

What is the difference between "assertive" and "aggressive"?

Becoming more assertive does *not* mean that a person becomes aggressive or bossy. Being assertive means honestly and openly expressing how *we* feel about something. They're *our* feelings. We're entitled to them. And we're also entitled to share them, not with the idea of forcing them on others but rather to let others know how we feel so they don't have to guess.

Being aggressive, on the other hand, expresses feelings but also usually incorporates being sarcastic, hostile, and putting others down. Aggressive people try to make others feel guilty and try to force their ideas, desires, and opinions on others. It's the difference between saying, "Why would I want to go to a stupid party and meet all those boring people?" (aggressive) and, "No thanks. I'd rather not go" (assertive).

It sounds simple, but for many of us, being assertive is difficult. We don't want to make people angry by saying no to something they want us to do—we think they may not like us anymore if we refuse—so we either say yes and find ourselves on a committee we don't want to be on or we make excuses.

"I'd love to be on the committee but I'll be out of town," we lie.

"That's okay," our friend tells us. "You can do all the work ahead of time."

"Well," we continue desperately, "I'd like to say yes, but I'm having the inside of the house painted so we couldn't have meetings there."

"That's okay," says our friend. "You can meet at my house."

And on it goes with our making excuses and our friend pushing until we finally give in and say yes. How much easier it would have been to say, "No, but thanks for asking." You don't need to offer excuses. Just be assertive and use the best four-letter word there is: "No no!"

Assertiveness takes practice

I don't mean to make assertiveness sound simple. For many of us, it isn't. As a matter of fact, it can be very difficult. I know from firsthand experience. For years I was an assertiveness dropout.

My office is in my home and always has been, except for an unsuccessful six-month experiment downtown. When my five kids were small, it was convenient to be able to go into the study and work and yet be on hand when the children needed me. The problem was, of course, that everyone else knew I was there, too. Also, because I worked out of my home, most people didn't think I "really worked." They figured it was all right to interrupt me because I was "only writing."

My friends would listen to me bemoaning the fact that I had an article deadline the following Friday and was expecting houseguests that same week. They'd shake their heads sympathetically—and then ask if I'd mind babysitting their kids as long as I was home anyway, or if I would help them write an article for a club newsletter.

I now know that I felt angry—inside. But I wouldn't have dreamed of letting my feelings show. These were my friends. I couldn't tell them no. After all, what are friends for? So I ran extra carpools, rewrote speeches and newsletter articles, and even went to a style show (I'd rather clean windows), all because I didn't want to hurt anyone's feelings.

My priorities always seemed to come last. In fact, I wasn't even sure I *had* priorities. Since I didn't rate them very highly, obviously no one else did either.

I felt tense, angry, and frustrated that no one really appreciated my writing. I was mad at myself for being such a pushover, too. Long after an incident had passed, I'd play the scene over and over again in my mind, thinking what I should have said. I hurt—physically hurt—because my gut was tying itself up in knots. That was the time that my irritable bowel symptoms were the worst. I not only didn't know what I had, I also didn't understand what my lack of assertiveness was doing to me.

Fortunately, at that point in my life I took some action. I did three things that improved my self-confidence as well as my mental and physical health.

First, I saw my physician who, after checking me out carefully, diagnosed my physical problems as being irritable bowel syndrome.

Second, I signed up for a noncredit course in assertiveness training at our local university. Those six weeks were among the most valuable I have ever spent because I learned how to express myself verbally and how to speak up for myself, becoming assertive and feeling better for doing so. Of course, like many others who have trouble asserting themselves, I feared I would become aggressive. I didn't. That trait is still a long way away on the continuum.

Many community colleges, universities, churches, synagogues, women's clubs, and hospitals offer assertiveness training classes. I heartily recommend your taking them. If they're not available in your area, I've listed a few excellent books you might want to get from your local library or bookstore. But you can't just read them; you have to practice what they preach as well.

The third step in my "awakening" program was to meet regularly with a psychologist. I learned how to begin to share my feelings of frustration about not standing up for myself. There was a lot of talk and tears on my part. For the most part, he just nodded and listened. One thing he did say, however, has stayed with me. It made me far more receptive to the assertiveness training classes. I'd like to pass it along to you.

I don't remember what I had been talking about, but it had something to do with not feeling in charge of my life, feeling that I was only reacting and doing things for everyone but me. "I feel like a convenience store," I complained, "always available, twenty-four hours a day."

"Will those folks die for you?" he asked quietly.

Although it's been a number of years, I still vividly

remember being taken aback. "Die for me?" What did he mean? "Of course not," I answered.

"Then tell me, why do you let them live your life for you?"

I just sat there for the rest of my fifty minutes, thinking about that question. It really hit home. It changed my life. Only *I* could live my life and to do so, I had to take charge, to become actively involved in my life. I could no longer be content to sit back and let people draw on my good nature, siphoning off the precious hours of my day. I had to decide how much of me I was willing to share.

Of course, that also meant that I had to start taking risks, assuming blame when things didn't go right. I no longer could say, "I didn't have time to work today. I had to help Martha with her committee." The difference—and it was an important one—was that if I didn't work, it was *my* choice, because no one was forcing me at gunpoint to avoid the computer. If I offered or allowed myself to be talked into doing a task, I had to take the responsibility for doing so.

It worked. I no longer felt pressured into spending my time the way others wanted me to. I was choosing what *I* wanted to do and making that choice made me feel good.

Obviously, all of us do many things that we might not prefer as a first choice. We have to attend certain business meetings, go to social and civic functions when we'd rather stay home with a good book, or watch sporting, theatrical, or television events just because the person we love enjoys them and wants to share them with us.

But by learning to become assertive, you are able to serve on committees and work for organizations of *your* choosing, not your friend's. You can begin to feel comfortable saying, "No, I'd rather not write the newsletter, but I'd be happy to handle decorations." You can even attend events you find silly or boring, but enjoy being there because you chose to be there with your friend or mate.

Assertiveness helps you to run away

But it's more than speaking up to do things. When you can be assertive, you can also make the choice *not* to do things. Sometimes it's more comfortable to take flight, rather than fight.

Recently, I got into a battle with a television cable company. We were without service for three weeks, and although they sent out four different service people to fix it, none of them could find the difficulty. Each of them did, however, assure me that the charges for my days without cable would be subtracted from my bill. When the bill came, it was the usual charge with nothing deducted. By then, a fifth repairman had located the problem. The wire had been cut by the lawn mower.

You've all had the same runaround, I'm sure. It took four calls to get hold of the proper person, who then said he'd check and get back to me. Four more calls and he said he had located the mix-up. He promised the thirty-six dollars would be removed from my bill.

My intestines, which had been protesting right along with me, finally settled down—until I received the next bill. Only eighteen dollars had been credited to my account. I was angry. I was upset and I hurt. Then I remembered that assertiveness put me in control of my own decision-making. Right or wrong, precedent or not, I decided that it wasn't worth fighting anymore for eighteen dollars. The price I put on my sense of well-being was far higher. You may have continued the fight, but for me, at that moment in my life, it wasn't worth it. But *I* made the decision. I was in control.

How does assertiveness affect IBS?

Becoming assertive does give you more control over your life. You'll feel less passive and even when things don't go exactly as you'd like, when you've expressed yourself you can at least feel that you've "gone on record" or "said your piece." You've been heard from. You matter. Your self-image is bound to rise and the stress that comes with feelings of being used or taken advantage of will lessen. As your stress level lowers, you'll relax and your intestinal tract should begin to settle down as well.

It doesn't mean that you'll never suffer from another IBS symptom, of course. It's a chronic problem and as such will recur from time to time. But the discomfort should begin to come less often and, it is hoped, be less severe.

Time management lowers stress

Remember the White Rabbit in *Alice in Wonderland*? The poor thing was always late. No wonder he was so frazzled. Deadlines do create tension in most of us, probably because it's human nature to let things go to the last minute. Think back to high school or college and term papers. No matter how early the professor assigned them, the deadline always seemed to be somewhere over the next hill, as far away as middle age seems to a teenager. Then up it popped, and we burned the proverbial midnight oil trying to get tired fingers to type on the typewriter keys, not in the cracks between. Tension mounted—migraines, backaches, and stomach pains flourished.

Many of us still do live with deadlines, some self-imposed but nonetheless stressful. Learning to manage time is not some obscure textbook science, but rather a living skill that everyone should learn, especially those of us with IBS. The goal isn't to become obsessed with time and schedule each moment to its fullest. That only creates *more* stress than we already have. Instead, time management is really self-management. It teaches us to examine our priorities and to take control of our days.

Each of us has the same amount of time each week, just 168 hours. We can decide how to spend that time by making conscious choices. Determining priorities and making those choices gives us control over our lives, which can reduce stress. By now, we all know how stress adversely affects us.

When I decided to become a full-time writer, I had five children eight and under. I wondered where I'd ever *find* the time to write. I never did find it; I made it. I took time I had been spending other places and allotted it to my writing. It meant analyzing and changing priorities; it meant communicating with my family and not expecting them to read my mind; it meant eliminating some things I had previously done and, in some cases, hurting a few feelings because I was no longer willing or able to be "on call."

Put it in writing

List-making—as long as you don't spend unnecessary time recopying your lists so they look better—saves time and reduces the pressure of trying to remember everything. Albert Einstein said *he* never cluttered his mind with unimportant facts, so why should you? Lists also help a family to share responsibility. If you have a grocery list posted on the refrigerator, for example, everyone will soon learn that nothing gets bought if it isn't on the list.

Carrying and using a date book also saves you time because you know exactly where you should be and when. Having your dates visually displayed in writing will help you prevent scheduling too many appointments too close together. Enjoy seeing the white space between meetings. Allow for traffic delays and unexpected phone calls.

The type of date book you use is extremely personal. I spent a half day in a stationery store trying to decide what would work best for me. Finally, I decided on two. There is THE BOOK, which shows a week at a time. I used to use a full month calendar, but it seemed overwhelming to see so many dates staring at me each morning.

Everyone in our family of seven uses THE BOOK to record their comings and goings. If it isn't there, it isn't happening. I list people's birthdays (with age, so I can remember the "important" ones), business trips, vacation time, social engagements, sporting events, doctor appointments (put the name of which child beside the appointment so you won't bring the wrong kid, as I once did), and my deadlines.

I also carry a small date book in my purse along with addresses and phone numbers. If you have two calendars, as I do, it's extremely important to remember to cross-check them each morning to be sure they have duplicate information. One special advantage of carrying a date book with you is that many people don't. It gives you a psychological advantage and also helps you control when meeting dates are set.

Reexamine priorities

Priorities, like our bodies, are ever-changing. Yet some people think of them as set in cement and create unnecessary stress by trying to cram their lives into molds that no longer fit. It's like wedging your size seven foot into a size five shoe. You might succeed, but not without a great deal of pain.

One man complained to me that he felt a great deal of stress because the minute he walked into the house after work, his wife insisted on his sitting down for dinner.

"Have you told her?" I asked.

"No," he replied. "She should know."

Many people share this opinion that those who know and love us should "know" how we feel about things. Yet mind-reading is not one of my skills. How about you?

I suggested he share his feelings about dinner with his wife. She was surprised, to say the least.

"But you *always* wanted dinner right away," she said. "You used to be angry when it wasn't ready."

He looked at her in amazement. "That was ten years ago when I was still taking night classes," he said. "I had to eat right away so I wouldn't be late."

Strange? Yes, but it's a true story. She had never changed her priorities and he had never communicated to her that it was time to reassess them. Their dinner hour is much more relaxed now that neither of them seems as rushed, and he claims to have fewer IBS flare-ups than he did in the past.

I learned to reevaluate priorities as my children moved out of childhood and into their teens and now, for all but one, into their twenties. The traditions that we all had loved and shared—making Christmas cookies, family Fourth of

July picnics at the beach, birthday cake at breakfast time—
all became more difficult as the kids grew and had their own
needs and priorities. Baking cookies became a chore at a
time when we all felt under stress anyway; the kids felt torn
between family loyalty on the Fourth of July and wanting
to be with their friends; nobody wanted to eat birthday cake
at breakfast anymore because everyone was dieting and we
all got up at different times.

By being assertive and honest about our feelings—you'll
find that as you become more assertive, the rest of your
family does, too—we slowly weeded out those traditions,
however wonderful, that no longer worked for us. It made
those we retained and the new ones we adopted that much
more special. By protecting our time and doing those things
that are meaningful to us all, everyone feels less stress and
enjoys those things we still do together—such as shorter but
still looked-forward-to family vacations, special dinners,
and silly gifts.

Check out your personal priorities, too. Are you still vac-
uuming every day although your long-haired sheep dog has
gone to the great doghouse in the sky? Do you still send
Christmas cards out to people you hardly remember? Are
you on the membership roster of more organizations than
you could ever really support? How much time do you spend
on the telephone and watching television each day? Keep
track of these potentially "terrible twos" in your detection
diaries. How many hours a day? How many hours a week?
These two specific time eroders may be the main reason
you're always running late.

Remember that you don't have to do everything yourself.
You can get help from your family or hire others to do it
for you. If you don't have extra money to pay someone, try
to barter services. You may hate to clean and love yard work
and find someone who's willing to trade chores.

Don't strive for perfection. Not only is it unattainable,
you'll drive everyone else crazy if you expect it and you'll
create stress and frustration in yourself. Many things just
need to be done; they don't have to be done perfectly.

Eliminate what doesn't need to be done so frequently, if

at all. Save your valuable time and energy for those things that have to be done and those things you enjoy doing.

Organization reduces "mess stress"

Where do you keep the dog's shot records? How old are those magazines stacked up, unread, in the corner? If the lights went out, could you find a flashlight that worked? Do you have clothes piled up on a chair in the bedroom?

Clutter, the mess we've all learned to love because it's ours, can and often does create a great deal of stress. It's especially bad when two people with different clutter quotients move in together. I'm speaking from firsthand experience here.

I have stacks of magazines and books marked with strips of paper balancing precariously on my bedside table like the boulders at Stonehenge. My husband's nightstand looks like something out of *House Beautiful*. My desk has that "used look," with pens, pencils, books, and articles layered two inches thick. His desk has a mug with freshly sharpened pencils and a notepad.

Fortunately, we've been together long enough that my clutter only makes him mutter now. But there have been times when I wasn't able to put my finger on a tax letter or cancelled check quite fast enough to keep his teeth from grinding. Before I began using color-coded file folders (red for medical articles, blue for general writing, green for money-related matters, etc.), I had been known to accidentally file bills in with manuscripts, where they languished for months, the bills unpaid and the articles unsold.

Clutter tends to multiply like wire hangers and can create frustration and added stress in your life. A little organization will make you feel much more in control. You don't have to become an efficiency expert with clipboard and stopwatch to become organized. Actually, it's fairly painless and gives a great deal of pleasure when you know exactly where something is because it's where it's supposed to be.

Without trying to make you feel compulsive about clutter,

here are a few general suggestions to help reduce your mess stress:

- When you see clutter (or have it pointed out to you), you have four choices:

  1. Leave it where it is
  2. Move it to another place
  3. Hide it so no one sees it
  4. Throw it away

- Curb collections. More possessions only mean more things to clean and store. Move collections behind glass so you can enjoy them without dusting them. If you have numerous collections, consider rotating them so only one is out at a time.
- Enlist the entire family to help control clutter. If you have small children, give them baskets and open shelves to hold their things. Lower hooks so they can reach them.
- If you're the messy one, try to figure out why. Are you trying to avoid responsibility? Get back at your mother? Don't want to take time to put things back?
- Buy duplicates. Have extra scissors, tape, and paper clips in each room where they're used.
- Think big. Throw out those tiny decorator wastebaskets and buy large ones so you're tempted to throw more away; the same goes for two-inch notepads by the phones.
- Give away cookware that only does one task, such as hot dog cookers, sandwich grills, etc., unless you have plenty of room to store them.
- Empty your closet of clothes you don't wear or that don't fit. When you buy a new blouse or pair of shoes, get rid of one that's old. You won't have to buy new hangers or enlarge your closet space.
- Have a "tidy box" and "dump it drawer" in each room so you can clean off counter tops. Eventually, of course, you'll have to empty these storage marvels, but with luck you can force yourself to throw away at least 20 percent of the things by then.

• Sort your mail over a large wastebasket. Throw junk mail out immediately unless you're sure you need it. Put bills in a bill box and have a special location for the rest of the family to find their mail.

Organizing your home and your life makes things less complicated. It should reduce some of the tension in your life. You won't find yourself with two meetings at the same time. You'll know where your car keys are. You'll always have ingredients for a quick meal in the pantry. You become in control, reducing both stress and the frequency of your IBS symptoms.

As you become more organized, you'll begin to find ways to productively use waiting time. Some people use those moments to practice relaxation. You'll find many techniques discussed in Chapter 13. Others bring a book or magazine, stationery, or needlepoint with them so a delay in getting in to see a doctor or lengthy wait at the garage, hair salon, or kids' school doesn't become stressful.

A pediatrician became adaptive at time management when he realized that leaving his office during the height of rush hour was creating unhealthy tension for him.

"When I left the office at five-thirty," he said, "the traffic was so bad that it was bumper-to-bumper and I didn't get home until six-thirty. When I arrived, I was tired, irritable, and overstressed. I decided to stay at the office until six, which usually gave me a quiet and unrushed half hour to see extra patients, return phone calls, and clear off my desk. To my surprise, the traffic was much lighter by then and I still got home at six-thirty, but I had done so without the stress of driving in heavy and often erratic traffic. I also had lowered stress by getting caught up on my paper work and phone calls so I could start the next day refreshed."

There are hundreds of ways that you could begin to get in control of your life, organizing your time, stress, clutter, and personal commitments. You just need to start thinking about them. As with any new skill, it takes time and effort. It often seems a little strange at first to know that you're in command. But you are. And you'll begin to feel better because of it.

Many books are available to help you learn more about assertiveness and time management. You'll find them at your favorite bookstore or library. A few I have enjoyed include:

When I Say No, I Feel Guilty, by Manuel J. Smith, Ph.D., published 1975 by The Dial Press. It's also available in paperback.

Don't Say Yes When You Want to Say No, by Herbert Fensterheim, Ph.D., and Jean Baer, published 1975 by David McKay Company, Inc., New York. It also contains some excellent relaxation techniques.

How to Get Control of Your Time and Your Life, by Alan Lakein, published 1973 by Peter H. Wyden and in paperback by Signet. This is the classic time management book.

Getting Organized, by Stephanie Winston, published 1978 by W. W. Norton & Company. It's very practical and also available in paperback.

=== 10 ===

Sharing With Others

Most of us have been using speech to some degree since we were about fourteen months old. Yet when it comes to actual communication, many of us are still like infants, making sounds that we expect others to interpret correctly.

"You should have known how I felt." How often have you thought that? How often have you said it aloud?

Yet few people admit to being mind readers. Most of us need to be told, not just verbally, with words and tone of voice, but symbolically, through nonverbal clues such as touching, body language, gestures, eye contact, and spatial distance. These nonverbal cues often speak far louder than the words we say.

Think about the person saying, "Trust me," as he refuses to look you in the eye and shifts uneasily from foot to foot, or the one who says she's interested in what you're saying, then looks at her watch, plays with her hair, and looks around the room to see who else is there. What are these people saying to you by their actions? How important are their words? Which speaks louder?

Foggy messages create stress

Without proper feedback, the speaker—parent, lover, teacher or boss—has no idea if the message given is the one received. Sometimes the mix-up can have disastrous results, as when the sergeant told the private to have the captain's horse "shod," and the private shot it.

When you waste an entire day doing an assignment wrong because you misunderstood your boss's instructions, when your teenager misses dinner and thought he'd told you he'd been invited out, or when you arrive an hour early for an appointment because you misunderstood the time, you're bound to feel frustrated, angry, and tense.

Your stress level may also rise when a person nods as though he or she understands, but when asked to repeat instructions, gets them wrong. Or when you're speaking to someone and can tell from the blank expression on her face or her glazed eyes that she's really not listening.

You can continue to stew in these situations and make yourself more uncomfortable, possibly triggering your IBS symptoms because of the added stress, or you can use the assertiveness techniques you've learned and tell the other person how you feel, saying that it bothers you when she doesn't listen. You also might tune in to what you're saying as well to see if maybe you do stretch a story out just a little too long with "he said . . . ," and "then she said . . . ," or too much detail. If people tend to shift attention while you speak or you're interrupted often, ask someone close to you to tell you if you ramble. It's often hard to hear ourselves. (If you're female, however, remember that many studies show that men tend to interrupt women more often than they do their own sex.)

Communication is a two-way exchange

Communication is not a one-way dialogue or monologue. True communication is a process, an interaction between a speaker and the listener. The latter has the obligation to give clues—verbally or through body language—that he or she is receiving the message, even if it's only a "hummm" or an occasional nod. The speaker needs to reinforce through feedback that the message given is the one received.

When someone talks to you, give them your full attention as well. Listening is a skill that we all need to develop more fully. Practice giving feedback, such as "Then you think we should redo the project because . . ." or "I know you want to have a later curfew and I understand your reasons. But I'd like you to listen to mine . . ."

Communication, like many things, gets better with practice. Marriage counselors say that most couples coming in for help have problems in one or more of three areas: sex, finances, and communication. Of the three areas, communication is probably the most important, because if a couple can learn to communicate and really listen to one another, the other two problem areas may be easier to work out.

Studies on stress in the work place often point to lack of communication between management and the labor force as a major problem.

Coping with mixed messages

Every communication has two levels of meaning: what is meant and what is actually said. We can say, "You've done a great job," or "Of course I'd like to," both of which sound like positive statements. Said with sarcasm or specific body language, however, both remarks can have very negative content.

Being on the receiving end of such mixed messages can be very confusing and frustrating. The meaning is distorted and you can become very tense trying to decipher what the speaker really was trying to say.

If you catch yourself giving these mixed messages, try to consciously think out what you're trying to say and communicate an honest message. If you're on the receiving end, practice your assertiveness (see Chapter 9) and tell the speaker you don't understand what he's trying to say.

If you're unlucky enough to have a boss that sends mixed messages, don't passively accept the tension that is bound to build up as you wonder where you really stand. Ask for a conference and assertively and comfortably ask for a "translation." It may be possible that your boss wasn't aware of the mixed message.

Families have a special language

Most families develop unique forms of communication as they grow and develop. There may be "inside jokes" or "code words." Family members may have nicknames used only within the family grouping and never in the outside world. Since their experiences are similar, family members often talk in abbreviated language. Difficulties and tensions may arrive along with in-laws or stepfamilies; they often feel left out because they don't, as yet, understand the language.

Each family is unique unto itself. Thus, there is no one "right" way for members to communicate within their family unit. It is true in most families, however, that each member quickly learns the "fuse point" of every other family member. That's why your sibling can "get to you," in a way no one else can. He or she knows your fears and your weaknesses.

Often, the tension that arises during gatherings of the clan comes from the knowledge that you are vulnerable. While you may feel a special security gained from the comfort of your family circle, you also are fully aware that all your foibles and failings may be spread out at the dinner table along with grandma's best cloth.

Family issues also trigger stress

Because of the closeness of a family, what affects one member also can create great stress among the others. Disagreements over life-styles, a chronic illness, the death of a family member, divorce, or the merging of families through marriage can all create change in the family dynamics and trigger stress. In fact, the first twelve events listed in the Holmes-Rahe Social Readjustment Rating Scale (see Chapter 4) create major role changes within the family structure.

Learning satisfactory communication techniques can be most helpful in reducing the stress created by the many changes experienced by a family. This skill, along with others you have read about in this book—such as assertiveness, time management, relaxation, and exercise—can be instrumental in providing an atmosphere conducive to family harmony. With open and honest communication, you should be able to reduce the tension level in your home, a goal desired by everyone, especially the IBS sufferer.

Many churches and synagogues, colleges, mental health professionals, and social organizations conduct workshops for families, covering such issues as decision making, fair fighting rules, family meetings, how to improve communication skills, and the art of listening. There also are many good books on these subjects in libraries and bookstores.

Talk to a friend

There's something special about a friend. A true friend, an entity as hard to find as Diogenes' honest man, is someone who accepts you, warts and all. You can unload your problems and fears to your friend, knowing that he or she will not pass them along. A true friend can be your mate or significant other—in fact, it's very special when the one you love is also your "best friend"—or he or she can be a co-worker, former classmate, neighbor, or someone you've met along the way. Your true friend's sex is not important, nor his or her sexual preference. What matters is that your friend be there for you and you for your friend.

Sharing your dreams, worries, and ideas with a friend is, like love, a bit of a risk. Your friend may not be loyal and may breach your confidence. He or she may drift away. You may, like lovers, fight and then make up. But having a good friend to talk to is an excellent stress preventative. You really do get tension off your shoulders.

"I always feel better when my buddy and I get together for a 'bitch session,' " said a secretary. "He's an accountant with another firm, but when we're together, we're on the same wavelength. I love him—as a friend—and we share information about parts of our lives that no one else knows about. *I* know he lacks self-confidence, although others think he's brimming with it. He knows I'm really shy. When I've had a tough day, I feel better telling my friend about it. He makes me laugh. When something good happens to me, it's not official until he knows. He makes me relax, feel good about myself, and smile. I smile a lot when I'm with him.''

Although to my knowledge, no studies have been done on the effects of close friendships on the frequency and severity of irritable bowel syndrome, I would speculate that maintaining a close friendship (with a spouse or friend) could have beneficial effects. Those with IBS often also suffer from depression and report stress from everyday worries about family relationships, problems at work, and numerous additional concerns that others might consider minor.

Having a close friend to share your feelings with should reduce that stress, providing you don't overload your friend with all your troubles and reenforce them in your own mind. I base this conclusion not on formal research but on personal experience, as well as on comments from over a hundred interviewees.

A few of these people said their "best friend" was their dog or cat. They reported that their pet was loyal, listened, and gave support back through licking or brushing up against them. It's really not so strange. Numerous studies have shown that a person's blood pressure can be lowered as he or she strokes and interacts with a pet. Most of us talk to our dogs or cats as though they were real people. But then, they *are*, aren't they?

Get to know co-workers as individuals

One problem area for many IBS sufferers is job-related stress. It can come from the job itself—it could be too structured or too unstructured, too difficult or too easy, or could take place in a poor working environment, such as crowded and noisy offices—or from difficulties interacting with other employees.

While other forms of action are needed to solve stress-related problems with the office environment and the job itself, better communication may ease the problem with co-workers. Often we work side by side in an office with people for years without knowing anything about them as people, individuals with dreams, worries, and ideas just like us. While you don't want to know everyone's life story, it can ease tensions when you begin to share a little of yourself with your co-workers and they begin to open up to you.

Obviously, you don't want to tell a co-worker the same confidences you would your best friend, nor should you tell anyone you work with anything you wouldn't want spread around your workplace. But it's easier to understand a co-worker's foul moods when you know that she just put her mother in the hospital or that her car was demolished by someone with no insurance. You can share the workload temporarily with someone when they've shared the news that they have serious problems at home.

Opening up to your co-workers and showing them a glimpse of your frailty, just as you begin to understand them as unique individuals, adds a touch of humanity to your office or workplace. It creates warmth, humor, and a sense of caring that is bound to reduce tension even in a stress-filled commercial climate where time is money and bottom lines are king.

Professional help is available

Some people just can't bring themselves to talk of personal matters to others. "I wasn't brought up that way," one woman said. "I wish I could, but I can't."

Another mentioned that she had been unable to share her thoughts ever since a friend betrayed her confidence by telling others what had been for the friend's ears only. Now she, like many others, held things inside and by doing so triggered a great deal of unnecessary stress.

If you have difficulty talking about what's bothering you, don't keep it bottled up. There is a wide network of professional people trained to listen in confidence, to help you make decisions about different matters or to help you just feel better for sharing your thoughts with someone else.

Some people feel comfortable talking with their religious leader. Those who don't or who have no religious affiliation may find a ready ear at a mental health clinic (freestanding or connected with a hospital) or with a psychologist, psychiatrist, social worker, nurse, or other therapist who is licensed to listen and help you reflect, and who may make suggestions to make you feel better, not only about yourself, but about the situation bothering you as well.

You are never alone. There are many people who want to help and who can help. But you need to speak up for yourself and let them know you need support. Don't be too proud to ask for assistance. All of us, at some point in our lives, have felt depressed, have thought we couldn't handle everything on our plate, have needed a shoulder to lean on.

Talk your way out

Stress is the natural reaction when too many events crowd in on us at once and we feel unable to cope. With changes coming so quickly in today's world, many of our learned responses are no longer effective. Everything seems different. New technology makes us feel stupid when we can't operate a simple VCR and our seven-year-old can. Computer literacy seems to be making library cards obsolete; marriage and child-rearing patterns are varied; manners and morals have no absolutes. Learning to adapt and cope in this new world is a must.

Effective communication, the skill which allows us to reach out to others, is, as with so many other skills, greatly improved with practice. It offers almost immediate rewards, not the least of which is reduction of stress. If you doubt that, just remember the smile on a tourist's face when he meets someone who speaks his language.

So don't wait. Work on improving your communication skills today and start sharing yourself with others. Come on in. The water's fine. And we're all in this great big pool together.

11

Talking To Yourself

I used to think I was a little crazy when I talked to myself. After all, didn't my teachers used to say, "Only sick people talk to themselves!" and "He who talks to himself talks to a fool!"

But they were wrong. When I began to devise ways to reduce the stress I felt, I unconsciously began talking to myself . . . often out loud. And I discovered that it worked. Why shouldn't it? After all, who knew me better than I did myself? Who knew what I was feeling better than me?

When I found myself procrastinating, tense with doubts concerning my ability to handle a particular writing assignment, I turned cheerleader. Interrupting negative thoughts of, "I've never done this type of writing before," I told myself, "Of course you can. And if you can't do it, no one can!" I reminded myself of all the other work I had done successfully. Once again, I felt in control.

When I felt frantic and pressed for time, and recognized the familiar gut-gripping signals of impending IBS problems, I turned traffic cop and arrested myself. "Okay now, what's the hurry? Slow down, you'll get more done. There's plenty of time if you just take it easy." I stopped and listened to myself. It made sense. I slowed down and did get more done because my body wasn't struggling with itself to do ten things at once. I was relaxed and focused. Everything was in harmony. What's more, I felt better.

Some experts, who probably don't want to go on record

telling people it's okay to talk to themselves, prefer to call it "self-verbalization." It really doesn't matter. What's important is that we do it and that we listen to ourselves.

What's the worst that can happen?

Usually we create unnecessary stress on ourselves by "pyramid thinking," that is, piling one imaginary thought on top of another until the teetering stack of problems is overwhelming.

It goes something like this: "I have to write this proposal for my boss and I don't know where to begin. Even if I do write it, it probably won't be any good. Even if it's good, it won't be strong enough to help us get the account. And I don't know where to get the information . . ." Well, you see how it builds. What usually happens is that we so overstress ourselves with this fear of failing that we procrastinate and never get anything done. Stress has made our fear of failure a self-fulfilling prophecy.

Perhaps we worry about how we look, whether our suit or dress is appropriate for a particular function. "I don't want to be overdressed. But I don't want to be too casual either. Everyone will be looking at me. I'll feel self-conscious . . ."

We build up so much tension agonizing over our outward appearance that we either make ourselves feel rotten and skip the whole affair or we go, but are under so much stress that we don't enjoy ourselves.

The truth is, unless you really look totally out of place—if you wear shorts at a formal cocktail party or a long sequined gown at a business seminar—chances are no one will really notice what you're wearing. If they do, and it's different from what *they* chose, it's possible they'll think *they* selected the wrong outfit, not you. You're not the only insecure person in the world, you know.

Speaking in front of large groups brings out insecurity in most of us. Although I enjoy the actual act of public speaking, the pre-terror used to cause me real pain. It didn't just trigger my IBS symptoms, it exploded them! I felt my intestines turning to ice water and experienced cramping, bloating, and diarrhea. I asked myself, "*Why* am I doing this? Why did I say, 'yes' when they asked me?"

Then I learned how to talk to myself. "What's the worst that can happen?" I'd ask.

"Well, I can forget what I'm talking about."

"Is that likely?" I'd ask myself.

"Well, no. I know the subject fairly well."

"So what's the worst that can happen?"

"I may bore the audience."

"What if you do?" I'd ask myself. "What's the worst that can happen?"

Eventually, I'd admit to myself that it was highly unlikely that any audience would throw their leftover chocolate pudding at me—and even if they did, I was three-fourths hidden by the podium. It also was quite unlikely that anyone in the group would boo me. The worst that could happen was that they would get up and walk out. And if that was the worst that could happen, I agreed that I could live with it.

By the time I completed this self-dialogue, I couldn't help but notice that my guts were calming, my pain was gone, and I was breathing more normally. Without having to enlist the help of anyone else to hear me out, I'd talked myself into a less stressful state.

Talk yourself through a situation

Remember those movies in which the pilot passes out and the only one left to land the plane is a sweet young thing who's never flown before? Somehow she manages to get the radio working and the handsome young man in the control tower "talks" her in.

"A little more to your left," he says. "Pull up. That's good."

"I don't know if I can . . ." she stammers.

"You're doing fine. Just fine," he purrs. By this time, you've probably dozed off, but the bottom line is, the girl lands the plane because *he* makes her think she can do it.

You can do the same thing for yourself. Well, perhaps

you won't land a plane, but with practice, you should be able to talk yourself down from tension and land into a state of calmness. You already know how to talk to yourself. Think about it.

You're learning to play golf. You stand ready to tee off. What do you say? "Check my grip, head down, left elbow straight . . ." Eventually, with practice, you'll do all that automatically, but as a novice, you're talking to yourself.

Have you ever taught anyone to drive? What do you say? "Adjust the seat, check the rearview mirror, fasten your seat belt. Okay, now insert the key . . ."

We all learn through self-verbalization, talking ourselves through each step until it becomes automatic. It doesn't matter if it's baking a cake, learning to water ski, mastering a new software program for the computer, or developing relaxation techniques. The process is the same:

1. Have the desire.
2. Learn the techniques
3. Believe you can do it
4. Practice
5. Keep practicing until you have mastered it

Comfort yourself

Four of my five children are of college age or older. The law states that they're adult now. They can vote; they can drink; their signature is legal without my cosigning. Yet whenever any of them are sick—with a high fever or flu, or another complaint—they want me to comfort them.

I can't blame them. Recently I was out of town and became quite ill. I wanted my mommy too! Medics during wartime admit that most of the seriously wounded fighting men they saw, no matter how brave and how macho, called out for their mothers.

We all need cuddling and comforting, regardless of how old we are. If we're fortunate, we have a spouse or close friend who can comfort us. But we can learn to comfort ourselves, too.

Talking aloud to yourself—or even speaking silently if you feel too weird talking aloud—can be extremely calming. Our vocal pattern is both familiar and soothing, like a mother crooning to a child. That alone, no matter what we are saying, is comforting. It doesn't matter whether it's a prayer, special phrase, or mantra; we concentrate on the sounds we are making and therefore are unable to focus on anything else. Also, while we're busy comforting ourselves, we forget to worry.

Oscar Hammerstein was right on target when he wrote the song, "Whistle a Happy Tune," for Anna in the hit musical, *The King and I*. Anna, a young widow, has just gotten off a ship from England. She and her young son have arrived in Siam, where Anna is to teach all the king's children. She is terrified, but as she explains to her child, when she whistles she can begin to talk herself into feeling confident.

It works. I don't whistle, but I've talked myself into a sense of confidence many times. You can, too. When you tell yourself everything is going to be okay, stand tall, and *look* sure of yourself, you soon begin to feel that way, too. After all, you wouldn't lie to yourself, would you?

I learned how successful this technique can be from one of my sons. He loves baseball and has played it since he was seven and slugged the ball off the batting tee. Now he plays high school ball. Although he's usually a fairly good hitter, in a recent game he struck out twice in a row.

"Are you nervous about batting again?" I asked him after the game.

"No," he shook his head. "Why?"

"Well," I answered, trying to be diplomatic. "You *did* strike out twice in the last game."

"I don't think about my strikeouts," he answered. "When I step up to the plate, I remember my hits."

Sometimes your kids amaze you! He's right, of course. Everyone makes mistakes. It's very human. We all strike out many times in life. But keep talking to yourself, reminding yourself of your successes. Visualize yourself as a winner.

Words can change feelings

When we were kids, we may have shouted back at bullies, "Sticks and stones can break my bones, but names can never hurt me."

It may have made us feel better saying that, but the truth is, names *can* hurt. I know men who don't dance socially because some unfeeling girl told them in high school that they were clumsy, and they bought into it. I also know people who have terrible physical pain because they've made some poor financial decisions and it keeps eating at them. They won't forgive themselves or give themselves permission to be human, to make mistakes as all mortals do. They feel they're stupid.

"Are you stupid about everything?" I asked one man who admitted his IBS symptoms were triggered after a long remission because he was "stupid" and made some poor investments in the stock market.

"No, of course not," he said.

"Just about financial dealings."

"No. I'm usually good in business," he said. "I just was too heavily into the stock market."

I asked him why he didn't give himself permission to make a mistake. "You'd accept a friend making a mistake in judgment without calling him 'stupid,' wouldn't you?"

He admitted that was so. Yet he had triggered real pain in himself by being much harder on himself than he would have been with someone else. By talking to himself and choosing his words carefully—calling his mistakes an "error in judgment" rather than proof of his "stupidity"—he was able to reduce his stress level and, soon, his physical discomfort.

The words you say to yourself can mold your world. Saying, "I'm so irritated by . . ." gives a different feeling than, "A funny thing happened when . . ." *You* feel differently when you tell yourself, "That was so dumb of me . . ." rather than, "Now that was silly . . ."

Treat yourself kindly. Speak nicely to yourself and listen. Words are symbols, and as such can trigger tremendous emotion. Words can soothe or they can be like acid and eat at everything (and everybody) in the way. You have the power to choose.

Shakespeare knew the power of words. "There is nothing either good or bad, but thinking makes it so."[1] We can give ourselves a boost toward a successful venture or talk ourselves into tension, stress, and failure. You may have heard the saying, "He's programmed himself for failure." It can happen.

When I first graduated from college, I wanted very much to get a job as a writer. They were difficult to find. A friend told me about an opening with a catalogue company, writing ad copy. It sounded perfect. I called for an interview, got one, and received directions on how to get there. It involved changing trains twice.

I began talking to myself, but in a negative mode. "What if I take the wrong train? How will I know when to get off? What if I can't find the company once I'm in that part of town? What if I'm late?"

Needless to say, I made myself so nervous and full of doubts that I was convinced I'd never find the place. I never even tried. I also didn't cancel the interview and have often wondered where that road would have taken me if I hadn't talked myself into failure before I even began.

Sometimes you can talk so negatively to yourself that you throw yourself—literally. Bonnie had done a good job for her company, so good in fact, that she was to receive an award at the monthly staff meeting. It meant leaving her place in the audience, coming up to the stage, and shaking the president's hand as he handed her the plaque.

"I'll never be able to do it," she moaned. "I'll trip. I know I'll trip. I can't possibly walk up those steps without falling, even if I wear low heels." She convinced herself, all right. She waited for her name to be called, walked to the steps, and tripped on the second step.

We're really a great deal like computers. We do what we're programmed to do.

Fool yourself

What we need to do is reprogram our destructive thinking. Put in a new "believe in myself" program. Just as you can talk yourself out of doing things, you can talk yourself into doing them. Erase the childhood tapes you may have been listening to, such as, "There's no use trying to do that, dear. You're not any good at it," or "Don't eat spicy foods. They always make your stomach hurt."

Create new tapes by talking to yourself and sending the messages you want to hear. Practice telling yourself, "I'm going to slow down and just concentrate on this one project. The others can wait," or "It's okay to say no to that committee job. I really don't want to work on it," or "I'm going to relax and enjoy this lovely meal. I'm in no hurry."

Sometimes it helps to have visual ticklers. I have a small turtle figurine on my dresser. I can't help but see it when I'm getting dressed in the morning. To everyone else, it's a cute little blue turtle. To me, it's a subtle reminder to "slow down." I see it, smile, and begin to breathe more slowly. After all, the tortoise won the race, didn't he?

I also have a visual tickler in my study, right by the telephone. I took a label maker and printed out the words, "Be realistic about your commitments." That label, in blue, stares up at me when I'm on the phone and whispers in my ear when I'm hesitating and may be about to say yes to another commitment.

Talk your anger away

Talk to yourself to reduce the stress that comes from the emotion of anger. Many people who wouldn't think of abusing their bodies with tobacco, drugs and alcohol, or junk food do just that by staying mad at the world. Within the confines of their car they shout abuse at other drivers. They yell at their kids, complain about service in restaurants and stores, and are sure that everyone in the world is out to get them. They're always in a fighting stance, ready to take on anybody they think is in their way. Then they wonder why their head hurts, their neck aches, and their intestines feel as though they're on fire.

But it doesn't need to be that way. Just as you can talk yourself into a good fight, you can also talk yourself out of one. Don't get mad, get relaxed. When you feel yourself getting angry at someone or a situation, don't see red. See green. Whisper "green" to yourself and allow yourself to picture springtime, with baby lambs cavorting all over a grassy meadow, flower buds poking up out of the ground, and soothing green fields with beautiful green trees swaying gently, back and forth in the wind. Whisper "green" and smell the scent of freshly cut grass. Hear yourself saying "green" and defuse your anger and its accompanying tension. Listen to yourself.

Discover the magic of laughter

Nothing breaks up tension as much as the sound of laughter. It's hard to stay angry, even at yourself, when you know the situation has a funny side, too. Tell yourself to look for the funny side of the street. It soon becomes habit-forming.

Numerous studies have shown how a sense of humor reduces stress. In his book *Anatomy of an Illness*, Norman Cousins describes how he feels laughter played an important part in his recovery from a serious illness. Laughing not only makes you feel good, it actually is good for the body, bringing additional air into the lungs, triggering healthy chemicals to flow through our system, reducing blood pressure and muscle tension, improving blood circulation, and reducing pain and depression. The power of laughter is now being seriously studied by researchers at many medical facilities. It must be good for us. Think about all the elderly comics we still have with us. Laughter certainly was good medicine for them.

One last note on laughter. The old saying, "Smile and the world smiles with you," is true. Test it for yourself by walking down the street or in a shopping mall and smile at people. Chances are, many will smile back at you.

Charles Spencer (Charlie) Chaplin, who probably knew

as much about laughter as anyone, said, "Laughter is the tonic, the relief, the surcease for pain."

Stop taking yourself so seriously. Learn to laugh at yourself and you'll feel so much better for it.

Never underestimate the power of the mind. You can talk yourself into calmness and into successful action. Like the little train that said "I think I can," you can use words to help motivate a less qualified team to outplay itself and beat the more skilled opposition; you can often talk yourself through pain, as women do in natural childbirth; you can beat down stressful feelings.

Words *are* magical, but it is *you* who is the magician. You put meaning into the words you say to yourself. Be kind to yourself and only say those words that help you to relax, to be in control of yourself, to succeed in those things that are important to you. Those "mind messages" are yours to create.

You're right if you're thinking that talking to yourself sounds a great deal like a form of self-hypnosis. In a way, it is. You'll learn more about that particular way to reduce stress in Chapter 13.

12

Discovering Personal Relaxation Techniques

While stress does not cause irritable bowel syndrome, there is a general agreement among the experts that it can and does trigger the symptoms. According to Drs. Marvin M. Schuster and William E. Whitehead, "It is important to note that the symptoms of IBS frequently occur in situations that are not objectively stressful (i.e., are not stressful for most people), but which may be associated with subjective anxiety for the patient with IBS.[1]

The detection diaries (described in Chapter 7) may help you determine those situations which are stressful so you can avoid or, at least, minimize them. In some cases, you may require the help of a psychiatrist, psychologist, or other mental health professional to help you understand how to cope with situational stress.

While it would be wonderful to be able to list everything you should do to help you relax and ease tension, that is impossible. Each of us is an individual and therefore each person must determine what works best for him or her. It's a trial and error effort, at best. Once again, one person's relaxation may bring real tension to another.

When I moved to a new neighborhood a number of years ago, I was welcomed into the local garden club group. It met infrequently, but when it did, each member was expected to present some type of floral arrangement.

My thumb is far from green. Not only do sweet potatoes fail to sprout for me, but I even lose leaves on plastic plants.

The approaching date for the garden club meeting filled me with real anxiety. Although I didn't realize it then, that stress triggered my IBS symptoms and I was too sick to attend the meeting. Despite my discomfort, I was delighted to have a reason to avoid showing my total lack of ability when it came to flower arranging.

Fortunately, I eventually was able to figure out that the only thing that grew for me in the garden club was anxiety, and that it obviously wasn't good for me. I resigned from the organization and felt embarrassed by the sense of relief it brought. Yet for another person, the garden club might have offered—and did for many—a tremendous sense of enjoyment and relaxation.

Pursuing the relaxing hobby

Most dictionaries define the word *hobby* as a pursuit done outside one's occupation for relaxation or pleasure. The key, of course, is the words "relaxation or pleasure."

Some people consider sports to be their hobby, but putt as though their life depended on the outcome or serve as though the object of tennis was to cram the ball down the opponent's throat. Although more discussion of the dangers of stress induced through sports can be found in Chapter 15, look in your detection diaries for times when you suffered from IBS symptoms soon after "relaxing" on the golf course or tennis court.

There's nothing wrong with a sense of competitiveness. It is exciting, challenging, and makes you feel alive. But if your hobby makes your heart pound with anxiety rather than aerobic exercise, your mouth and throat grow dry, and your guts churn, if it makes you tense and angry when you don't win, it isn't relaxing. It may bring you exhilaration, but it won't bring you serenity, nor calm your intestinal tract.

What does? Fishing, for some. I know people who can sit with a pole in their hand for hours, watching the bobber float up and down on the waves and not really caring if a fish takes the bait or not. Their breathing is slow and even,

their facial muscles are relaxed, and they're comfortable—
at least for that period of time—with their lives.

Dare to try the unusual as well. Dr. Stephen Allen, Jr.,
son of author and entertainer Steve Allen, is a medical doctor
with a specialty in family medicine. He learned to juggle and
discovered that it helped him to reduce stress. The late per-
former Mary Martin and former football star Roosevelt Grier
were also known for their expertise in needlepoint. They both
reported it was effective in reducing stress.

Others can sit at the piano and play their tensions away.
They enjoy the sound of the music, the touch of the key-
board, the act of creating. Some are as good as professionals while others have only had a few lessons and fake the
chords. The musical expertise doesn't matter. The ability to
find something that is relaxing for you is what's important.

Many people say they find listening to recorded music
relaxing. I have a neighbor who treats himself to one new
compact disc of either symphonic music or opera each week.
He relaxes out in the sun as his mind drifts off and he shuts
out the sounds of lawn mowers and kids playing. It gives
our neighborhood a very classy sound.

His wife, a wonderful cook, tunes in to another sense to
help her relax. Her home is often perfumed with cinnamon
boiling in a pot on the stove or her special potpourri blend.
The scent makes you want to slow down, breathe deeply,
and dream of faraway gardens.

It may take trial and error before you find what unwinds
you and calms you. No one can do it for you, and what
relaxes your best friend or spouse may be stressful for you.
Keep searching.

Try crafts like needlepoint, knitting, and hooking. Play
with watercolors, oils, or charcoal. Experience the tactile
pleasure of kneading bread, stamp collecting, gardening . . .
the list is endless. Whatever you discover, it should be relaxing and give you pleasure. If it isn't easily accessible,
like riding or sailing, try thinking about it. Shut your eyes
and imagine yourself doing it. After a while, just mentally
picturing yourself engaged in your hobby should be enough

to relax you. You'll learn more about this process in Chapter 13.

The wonderful world of water

For most of us, being immersed in water is soothing. Perhaps it's a subconscious return to the womb where we floated around comfortably before being thrown out into this cold and crazy world.

Try using the bathtub as your private spa, what my friend calls her "immersion therapy." Tell the family you're claiming half an hour for yourself. If you have small children, get a sitter or trade off with a friend. This time's for you.

Turn the telephone answering machine on, ask others to answer the phone, or put a pillow over it so you won't be disturbed. (Don't take the receiver off the hook. The phone company claims it messes up the lines.) Fill the tub with bath oil or bubble bath and warm water. Don't make it too hot. Climb in and enjoy the sensation of the water all over your body. Shut your eyes. Breathe slowly. Enjoy the scent of the bath oil or bubbles. Relax. Let your toes bob up. Relax. If you've had gas or pain, you'll discover it easing as the warm water soothes and relaxes.

While you obviously can't hop into the tub in the middle of a major crisis at the office, you *can* relax yourself to some degree by remembering how the bubble bath felt against your skin and recalling its perfumed scent. You'll find your breathing slowing down and your body beginning to relax a little while you re-create the image in your mind.

Massage—that "hands on" feeling

Massage is defined as "the manipulation of the superficial tissues of the body, used for therapeutic purposes and stress reduction." It was used as far back as the ancient Greeks and Romans and has been used by the Chinese, Japanese, and other Eastern cultures for centuries.

Although there are different styles of massage, all involve

some degree of stroking and kneading the body. They vary according to the amount of pressure applied. Some massage, such as sport massage, goes deeper into the muscles to improve circulation and is more therapeutic in nature, working on specific problem areas. Swedish massage incorporates quick, invigorating strokes to the entire body.

I find my weekly massage to be vital in helping me to reduce my stress level. The weeks I can't fit it in, I can *feel* the difference. I'm fortunate in having a massage therapist who comes to my house with her specially constructed table. (Male practitioners are called *masseurs*, and females, *masseuses*.) I prefer having the lights low and the air conditioning off. She works for an hour, beginning with my neck (another tension spot for me), then continuing with my face, hands, arms, and down to my feet. I turn over on my stomach and she continues on my legs and back. When the time is up, I feel totally relaxed, yet filled with energy. (She says that's an unusual reaction as most people just want to fall asleep afterward.)

I don't fall asleep during the massage, either. But my mind is blank. I never remember thinking anything. I concentrate solely on the warm sensation of my muscles and enjoy the state of relaxation.

If you're thinking of trying massage for one type of personal relaxation, get references first, especially if the person is coming to your home. Check to be sure the person has been properly trained. Some states require licensing before anyone can work on clients.

Be sure to tell the massage therapist what type of massage you like. I prefer a deep muscle massage, but before I learned to be more assertive, I just lay quietly on the table feeling frustrated that the pressure wasn't hard enough. Some people prefer a light touch, almost a gentle stroking. If you have a massage in a spa or hair styling salon, there may be a lot of noise and the lighting may be regulated. If you have any choice, however, consider having the lights dimmed as it tends to lower distractions.

It may take you a few sessions before you know if you want music or silence. I hope you won't get a chatty massage therapist, as I once did in a resort. I didn't feel comfortable telling her to please stop talking despite the fact that I was paying for her service. (See, it's very stressful not being assertive!)

The young woman who is my regular massage therapist has been working with me for four years now. She recognizes my tension spots almost as well as I do. We chat a little as she works on my arms, but for the most part, I float relaxed in silence—just the way I like it.

Is having a massage a real luxury? To me, it's a necessity. I can skip the beauty shop—admittedly, I have short hair that doesn't need to be styled. I haven't had a manicure since my wedding day, twenty-seven years ago. I hang on to shoes until my regular shoe salesman begs me *not* to tell people they came from his store as many of them are four or five years old. None of these other pursuits does for me what an hour-long massage can do. It's a matter of personal taste, of course, but for me, massage is one of life's greatest inventions.

Daydreams take you there

"I'd love a massage," you wail, "but I'm in my office from nine to five and have meetings of one kind or another almost every night. How do *I* relax?"

Daydreams can take you there. You probably daydreamed as a kid in algebra or history class, but you probably got in trouble for it, too. While some people may not approve of letting your mind wander for a moment, most daydreamers say they feel more refreshed, stimulated, and renewed when they "come back to earth." According to researchers, daydreaming, for many people, is analogous to relaxation and meditation as it tends to relieve certain kinds of tension.

Dr. Thomas D. Borkovec, a psychologist at Pennsylvania State University, agrees that daydreams can be a pleasant form of brief relaxation. He adds, however, "Don't replace one habit (i.e., getting overstressed) with another. Don't get too removed. Daydreaming should never be used as escape, but rather as a brief release and respite."

With that warning to watch that you don't habitually retreat into fantasy, try dreaming your tensions away. Think of a favorite spot—at the beach, in the mountains, in the woods. See yourself relaxing or playing there. Tell yourself a story. Some people enjoy daydreaming as they listen to a favorite piece of music. Others open a box or jar of their favorite potpourri and let the scent carry them away. You might even try to emulate Linus in the "Peanuts" cartoon by stroking a piece of soft fabric, a smooth stone, or a pet. (Numerous studies have shown that stroking a pet can actually help lower blood pressure and reduce stress and depression.)

Try to utilize all your senses. Relax and dream away. You might outdo Walter Mitty.

How often do you see a tense cat?

While humans are supposed to be the most advanced species, I think we all can learn something about relaxation from the animal kingdom. Although I'm a dog lover, we have no dogs at the moment and have allowed my youngest daughter's two cats into our home—or perhaps it's they who have allowed us.

It's probably safe to say that most domestic "inside" cats (those whose declawed little paws have never touched soft grass or cold concrete) are not particularly tense creatures. Oh, they may panic a bit when they've wet on the new Oriental rug, but that's good sense, not tension.

They sleep a lot, draped precariously over kitchen cabinets or on backs of couches and chairs, or curled up in an empty grocery bag or magazine basket. I once opened a drawer, was distracted by the telephone, and when I returned, discovered Smudge, our twenty-two-pound neutered male cat fast asleep on the place mats.

Catnapping *is* a relaxing pastime. Many famous people—Winston Churchill, John F. Kennedy, and Thomas A. Edison, to name just a few—had the ability to drop off to sleep for a short nap and wake up feeling refreshed and totally alert. Many women report that their husbands are experts at catnapping, after dinner and in front of the television.

I have always envied that ability to doze. Those who have it say that it is a most successful and satisfactory way to reduce tension and that they feel far more relaxed when they wake.

If you have a cat, study it as it sleeps and watch how it stretches as it wakes. If you don't have one, call me.

Give yourself a bathroom break

"There's so much to do in the morning," complained a mother of three who suffered from IBS symptoms, especially constipation. "I don't have time to use the bathroom. After I've fixed breakfast and gotten all the kids off to school, I've lost the urge."

Ignoring the body's signals for a bowel movement is one of the major causes of constipation. Fortunately, it can easily be corrected. You simply need to retrain yourself, just as your mother trained you originally, by taking a bathroom break as soon as you feel the urge and letting nature take its course. Get up earlier, if necessary, so you'll have the extra time you need.

Give yourself that special time. You wouldn't rush a toddler during potty training or even a dog you were trying to housebreak. Why rush yourself? Relax by reading the newspaper or skimming a magazine. Turn the radio or stereo up so you can hear the calming music. This is *not* the time to listen to the news and hear the most recent terrorist activities, murders, or rapes. Relax. Close your eyes, if necessary, to shut out distractions.

When driving drives you crazy

For many people, it isn't the job that drives them crazy, it's the getting to work that does. Many of you don't have to do your own driving as you live in cities offering public transportation. While it frees you from having to drive to work, it also offers its own particular triggers for stress—

the feeling of being crowded, fears for safety, frustration from erratic schedules, and a sense of dependency on others.

Driving your own car, however, hardly frees you from those stresses. Most of America's roadways are jammed during what the broadcast industry terms "prime drive times" (six-thirty to nine A.M. and three to seven P.M.). Many drivers—not counting those already dangerous because they're under the influence of drugs or alcohol—resent being hemmed in by other cars or having to go to work at all, or just feel angry in general. The result is cars weaving in and out of traffic lanes, horns blaring, and blood pressures soaring.

I live in a major city and, as in most growing areas, find the highways filled with almost bumper-to-bumper traffic when I have to travel during prime drive times. For many years, I sat, a carbon copy of many other drivers—jaw set, teeth clenched, eyes narrowed, gripping the steering wheel until my fingers ached, and pounding the dashboard in frustration as the cars crept along like arthritic mice.

Then, when I began to use my detection diaries, I discovered that I often suffered from IBS pain and other symptoms shortly after I had been in one of those traffic jams. It didn't take a great deal of intelligence to realize that I was hurting myself by that situational stress.

What could I do about it? My office is in my home so I didn't need to drive to work. But often I did have meetings and interviews that required my being on the road at the same time everyone else was heading to work. I changed the appointment times whenever it was possible. When it wasn't, I altered my inner environment.

If you really think about it, each of us who drives is, in essence, sitting alone in a little podlike cell, racing—or more often, creeping—along the roadways completely self-contained, like an astronaut in a space capsule. Many of us have air conditioning, stereo and tape deck, everything but a TV and waterbed to make us feel completely at home. While we cannot control the traffic on the outside, we certainly *can* control the environment inside, and that's what I consciously decided to do.

I began to listen only to the classical music station on the radio and found the sound to be soothing and relaxing. My particular station is also free from continual commercial interruption, as they only schedule advertisements on the hour and half-hour.

I also bought a cassette tape of Robert Frost reading his own poetry and found that I so enjoyed and became so relaxed hearing Frost reciting "Birches," "The Death of the Hired Man," and "Mending Wall," that I never even noticed that my lane of traffic was hardly moving. More importantly, my intestinal tract felt as calm as I did.

A friend who claims to detest poetry of any kind purchased some of the "book tapes" now available and enjoys catching up on some of the best-sellers and yes, even the classics. It really doesn't matter what you're listening to—although I personally doubt that loud rock music relaxes anyone, including the kids who listen to it—as long as it keeps you from tensing up, leaning on your horn, and creating unnecessary stress.

Recently, I received a gift of over twenty tapes of "The Cinnamon Bear," a radio series from my childhood that I had loved. I put one on as I fought the rush hour traffic. I smiled with delight at hearing songs I hadn't thought about in more years than I care to count. I enjoyed myself so much I almost regretted the traffic jam breaking up so quickly.

I hesitate to admit that I also use a car phone, but I've had one for two years and find it invaluable, although expensive, for relieving stress. When I'm caught in a traffic jam, I can call ahead and say I'll be late; with the "hands off" device that allows you to speak while keeping both hands on the wheel, I can return necessary phone calls while I'm "wasting" time on the road. This allows me to come home and get right to work, rather than spending a half hour or more making phone calls and feeling upset that the day is getting away from me. If you haven't kept track of the time you spend on the phone, begin today. Log in when you pick up the receiver and log off when you hang up. If you're like many of us, you'll be horrified at the *hours* spent on the telephone.

If you can't or don't want to get a car phone, do invest in an old-fashioned egg timer for every telephone. For most calls, if you talk more than three minutes, you've talked too long.

Plan ahead

A study by Dr. Douglas A. Drossman showed that those with IBS often have symptom flare-ups during times of personal stress.[2] Although you may not be conscious of it, if you check your detection diaries you may find that symptoms tend to return to plague you, even if you've been in remission for a while, around the anniversary of a traumatic event such as loss of a parent or a divorce; around the Christmas holidays; on your birthday, especially if it's a "big" one (thirty, forty, or fifty) or the age at which one of your parents died.

With that advance knowledge, you need to try to clear your calendar ahead of time so you're not under extra stress and practice whatever relaxation techniques work best for you. If the Christmas holidays tend to get to you—and this more than any other time of the year seems to bring forth tension for most of us—minimize social events to those things you really enjoy, cut down on traditions that no longer hold meaning for you, and watch what you eat. Use your detection diaries frequently so you can discover what triggers your symptoms on "stress dates."

The secret, according to Dr. Thomas D. Borkovec, is in "tension cue identification." If you can learn to identify your personal stress cues and catch them early, you can use your choice of the many means of periodic relaxation to greatly reduce stress and its effect on your body.

====== 13 ======

Exploring Deep Relaxation Methods

Most of us come into this world with the gift of being able to relax whenever we get tired or overstressed. Infants and small children have the knack for dropping off to sleep or resting whenever and wherever they are—on the floor, on a parent's shoulder, or in the car.

But by the time we reach our teens, most of us have forgotten that spontaneous relaxation technique. We fight tension with tension, rather than allowing ourselves to grow limp and drift off. Fortunately, relaxation can be relearned. The procedure is called "progressive relaxation," and although the technique may vary slightly, depending on who gives the instruction, all versions are based on the same general principle.

Relaxation is the antithesis of muscular activity. If we're truly relaxed, we cannot be tense. Just as an athlete learns when to tense a muscle and when to relax it for ultimate performance during competition, we can learn through practice to relax our muscles to give us the greatest release from tension. This ability, however, doesn't come from a doctor's prescription pad or from a book. Reading about it does give you the basic information you need, but it won't do the job for you any more than reading a book on how to play tennis will make you a tennis player. The only way to learn progressive relaxation is the old-fashioned way, through practice and repetition until it becomes second nature to you.

The concept isn't new

Physiologist Edmund Jacobson is considered to be the "father" of progressive relaxation. More than forty years ago, he became convinced that prolonged tension could trigger certain illnesses. Jacobson felt that once a person became aware of muscular tension by consciously tensing different muscle groups, he or she could then be taught to reduce that tension. In 1929, he published a book describing his theories that was widely read by physicians and other mental health professionals.

Although progressive relaxation was a fairly new concept to the Western world, it had been practiced under different names in the East for many centuries. Early literature describes monks, rabbis, and other religious followers using various forms of progressive relaxation—called "yoga," "meditation," or "self-hypnosis"—to block out the cares and concerns of the physical world and focus on the spiritual side. Such techniques allowed the practitioner to achieve a state of tranquillity and peace in which breathing, brain wave activity, and heart rate slowed down and blood pressure dropped.

Much of this was achieved by retreating to a quiet spot, regulating breathing until it became slow and deliberate, and repeating some word or words on each outbreath. Recently, in the United States, people have paid large sums of money to receive their "special" mantra, but the specific word uttered really isn't that important. Its primary importance is to help focus the mind and prevent other thoughts from intruding. Actually, sometimes the word is merely a nonsense word or sound. Other times, it may have specific religious meaning or a significance only to the person using it.

What is progressive relaxation?

Progressive relaxation is a method of relaxation in which a person learns to recognize stress and muscle tension in his or her body, isolate it, and then reduce it consciously, transferring concentration to a word or phrase.

Although there are basically two forms of progressive relaxation—active and passive—they have the same goal: to create deep relaxation. In "active" progressive relaxation, you lie on a reclining chair, couch, or bed, slowly tensing and then relaxing different muscles in your body. Your mind directs your body to first tighten, then relax these muscle groups and feels the sensation that comes with relaxation.

Some techniques have you focus on a single word or phrase, while others may have you use imagery—visualizing being in a setting that suggests relaxation to you and imagining the smells, sounds, sights, and sensations of the location.

"Passive" relaxation is basically the same technique, but you don't tense your muscles first. Instead, you begin focusing on first your feet, then your ankles, working up to your face and scalp, relaxing the muscles in all areas.

Both techniques suggest you begin in a quiet place and practice at least once a day for ten to twenty minutes. Twice a day is even better, but most experts I talked with warned against more than that.

"The idea is not to withdraw from the world," said one, "but to be equipped to handle stressful situations by being able to relax and release the tension you feel."

Once you have learned to achieve deep relaxation in privacy, you then begin to transfer the same process to noisy and more stressful situations. The goal, of course, is to be able to achieve deep relaxation during times of stress when you really need it, not just when you're alone in the quiet of the bedroom.

What does progressive relaxation do?

Once it has been mastered, progressive relaxation can actually alter the chemical balance in your body, especially those chemicals triggered by stress, and, in some people, slow their irregular colonic activity. It can lower blood pressure and eliminate or reduce pain from headaches. According to Dr. Herbert Benson, author of the best-known recent version of progressive relaxation, called *The Relaxation Response*, it can also relieve nausea, diarrhea, and constipation. It is the proof that "mind over matter" is far more than just a saying. It works. That's why it is an important technique for anyone suffering from stress-related disorders to learn, and a vital and most welcomed skill for those of us with irritable bowel syndrome to master.

Jacobson recorded his success in using progressive relaxation to give relief to IBS patients in an article written in 1927.[1] Since that time, progressive relaxation used alone or in combination with other stress reduction techniques has helped many patients with IBS to improve greatly.

Where can you learn relaxation techniques?

Many people learn progressive relaxation or other relaxation techniques from their physician, a psychologist, a psychiatrist, or another mental health professional trained in their use. They work with the professional until they feel comfortable with the relaxation procedures and can produce the same effect on their own. If you need to find someone in your city, look in the Yellow Pages under "psychologist" or contact the Mental Health Department of your city or state.

Your library and bookstore probably have a great many books on various relaxation techniques, including yoga, imaging, and meditation. Most of them also contain examples of how to learn the procedure. The best one, in my opinion, is *The Relaxation Response*, by Herbert Benson, M.D. Originally published in 1975 by William Morrow and Company, Inc., it was later reprinted in paperback by Avon Books.

As it is impossible to read the directions for the various steps at the same time you try to put them into practice, you need to either enlist a friend to read them to you or tape-record the steps. Many commercial companies offer relaxation tapes for sale. Some are rather expensive and are meant more for a professional's use with patients than for a layman's personal use. As there are numerous relaxation-tape ads appearing in a myriad of magazines, there is no way to review them all.

My personal preference among the commercial tapes I have heard is a set of two tapes, one on passive relaxation by Dr. William Redd and one on active relaxation by Dr. Thomas Burish. At this writing, the cost of the set of two thirty-minute audiocassettes is $25. They may be ordered from:

Carle Medical Communications
110 West Main Street
Urbana, IL 61801-2700

After reading about progressive relaxation and other forms of relaxation, however, you may decide to write and record your own steps, incorporating your own style and also the scenes that may be relaxing for you. This is what I did.

I originally learned active relaxation from a psychologist who was most patient with me, as my mind tended to wander and unwanted thoughts kept popping in, like northern guests to Florida during winter. Everything was going well until he told me to picture myself flying and landing gently on a soft white cloud.

What he didn't know, of course, was that he was talking to a charter member of the frequently frantic fliers club. I'm so afraid of heights that I actually made my husband exchange our season basketball seats at the local university because our existing seats were so high up I couldn't bear to look down at the court. So, my first attempt to relax by picturing myself flying and landing on a cloud, fluffy or not, worked me up into a real anxiety attack.

After I finally mastered the technique, I went into business for myself. I wrote and recorded my own adapted version. It's me, talking to myself, but as that's what I do quite frequently (see Chapter 11), it works for me. I'm including a sample script at the end of this chapter. Remember, however, that it's written especially for me. You may need to adapt it so it works for you as well.

How to achieve deep relaxation

• **Find a quiet spot.** That, in itself, often presents a real challenge. If you have young children and there *is* no quiet spot in your home, you may have to be creative. Ask a friend if she'll babysit while you borrow her basement, guest bedroom, or living room floor, or make the kids' naptime your relaxation time. If you work, get up a little early or use your lunch hour. It may take about forty-five minutes in the beginning, but after that, thirty minutes should be plenty of time.

• **Get comfortable.** Find a comfortable chair or lie down on a couch or bed. Loosen your waistband, tie, or any other article of clothing that may be binding. If you wear glasses, remove them. Take off your shoes as well as any jewelry that may dangle against your body and disturb your concentration.

• **Close your eyes.** It helps me to picture a thick, dark black velvet curtain like a theater curtain behind the proscenium. It is completely black, and the pile of the velvet fabric is so thick you feel as though you can fall into it, falling gently, floating. (To my surprise, as I write this description, my face feels relaxed and numb and my eyes are heavy. These thoughts have drifted me into relaxation many times before. Now, my mind and body seem to find it natural to respond as they have been trained to do, not realizing that if they do, I'll never get this chapter finished.)

• **Let your mind go blank.** Try to let your mind go as blank as that dark velvet curtain. Don't try to "make" it blank.

Just drift as though you were in a rowboat on a peaceful lake—unless, of course, you hate boats or are afraid of water. The only word in your mind should be the word or phrase you have selected as your "mantra." It can be as generic as "love," "peace," or "calm." It also can be a word or phrase that has some spiritual meaning for you, such as "God," "Buddha," "Jesus," etc. It also can be a sound, such as "hmmmm," or "ahhhhh."

• **Let unwanted thoughts float by.** Picture yourself under an invisible umbrella, a plastic shield, or a glass dome. When your mind wanders—and it will—just think, "Float by." Let those extraneous thoughts bounce off your shield and float by. Let them drift away like those astronauts in the movies who lose their grip on the mother ship.

• **Move in your mind to a soothing scene.** Be careful to select something that is truly relaxing to *you*.

• **Be patient.** Don't become frustrated if it takes a while to learn relaxation. It's like any other skill you learn. You wouldn't expect to sit down at the piano after a few lessons and play a concerto, would you? Hardly. You'd begin with scales, then add chords, and practice a great deal. You'd expect to hit many wrong notes before you played the piece correctly. Deep relaxation is like that, so don't expect perfection or success immediately. Just keep trying and you'll make progress. Remember the tortoise!

When a raincoat gets dirty, you send it to the dry cleaner's to be cleaned. After they do so, they have to add a protective coating to make it waterproof again. Otherwise, it would absorb water like any other garment. Stress-reduction techniques are a lot like this water-repellent agent. They won't eliminate stress in the world any more than a raincoat eliminates rain. But both can protect you from getting soaked.

Relaxation reminders

Now you faithfully practice relaxation techniques once or twice a day until you can evoke relaxation at will. You have learned to unwind in your quiet, private place without much difficulty. But what happens at the office? In the subway? In a waiting room? Standing in line at the supermarket? When you find yourself in situations that your detector diaries warn are "problem areas"? How do you prevent stress from building up while you're in front of a classroom teaching thirty restless kids? When you're sitting at your desk in the midst of forty identical desks all lined up like West Point cadets while everyone is watching? Can you take off your shoes, loosen your waistband, and begin chanting your mantra? Obviously not. So what then?

You need to keep practicing the relaxation techniques until they become almost second nature and you can easily call up the response through personal cues or reminders. I use the car's windshield wipers as one of my subtle reminders. Even when it doesn't rain, I tend to bump them on each time I turn the key. I only let them flop back and forth a few times, but the motion reminds me to let myself drift to my private spot and conjures up a sense of relaxation.

The scene that is soothing to me is an old-fashioned rope swing hanging from a tree on top of a hill—not a very high hill. It overlooks a bay with sailing ships just on the horizon. I can almost see myself swinging back and forth on that swing and feel the gentle breeze blowing against my face. The smell of salt fills my head. I slowly breathe in and out, thinking "calm," "calm," with every exhalation. I think the motion of the swing reminds me of my childhood, when I had no sense of urgency about anything and could swing for hours watching a butterfly flit around the sandbox or seeing clouds form into shapes like pictures. To me it's soothing, relaxing, and means peace.

The flopping windshield wipers are my hint to return to my swing and feel the breeze. They're like a toddler peeking around the corner at the playground to make sure Mommy's still there. When she is, the little one can continue playing, relaxed in the knowledge that security is close by. It works the same with your private hideaway. Just checking every so often to make sure it's there can trigger relaxation in most people.

If you don't drive or use the car often enough to help you on a daily basis, create other reminders. Let the red traffic light be your hint to stop and relax. Pause for a few seconds when the phone rings to breathe in and out, slowly, as you let tension float by. Use a mirror or store window. Are you wearing a frown? Is your jaw set? Are your shoulders hunched? Are your hands clenched? Float to your spot and relax. Slowly breathe in and out. Passersby won't notice and if they do, they'll think you're looking in the store window.

Use your waiting time—at a doctor's office, in line at the post office, in a restaurant—to relax. If you sit in an office all day, have a special pencil that you can touch, and feel yourself growing relaxed as you float away in your mind for a few seconds. You can also use a flower or a figurine.

I collect hippos—figurines and pictures, not the real ones—and have a lovely stone hippo that sits on my desk. He feels like a cool worry stone. He's smooth, but has gentle curves. When I'm feeling tense and have to be at my desk, I stroke my hippo and hippotise myself into floating to my hilltop for a moment or two.

Some people require less subtle reminders to help them relax. Several people interviewed for this book reported using a metronome to tick them into feeling calm. One woman said that with each tick of the metronome, she could feel herself moving further and further back into the warm dark cave where she felt safe and at peace. Anyone with claustrophobic problems might feel as though she or he was being buried alive, rather than calm, but for this particular woman, it was her safe spot.

Relaxation reminders are as individual as people themselves. Some of the suggestions I've gathered from others include these:

• Take your watch off and each time you glance at your bare wrist, take a moment to relax.
• Post a "relax" sign on the telephone.
• Hang a mirror by the phone so you can check your tension level as you talk.
• Practice relaxation during commercials on television.
• Get an aquarium for your office and each time you feel

angry or frustrated, follow the movements of one of the fish for a while.

* Take an extra few minutes in the bathroom to close your eyes and relax.
* Count backwards from ten, slowly, every time you look at a clock or your watch.
* Ask someone to remind you to take a "relaxation break." Long before I had ever heard of relaxation procedures, I was working with a friend on a project. At four, she called home to her teenage son and asked him if he had remembered to practice his relaxation. At the time I thought it was a little strange. Now I realize how lucky that youngster was to learn to evoke relaxation at such an early age.

Others have mentioned using recorded sound as their reminder. You can buy or make tape cassettes of waterfalls, gentle rain, ocean breakers, or water fountains. Some people prefer using musical cues. It's really a very personal choice.

For me, sound is an intrusion when I'm really trying to concentrate—either on writing or on relaxing. One evening my masseuse brought a tape recording along when she came to give me a massage. "A lot of my clients find it relaxing," she said. I had my doubts, but was willing to give it a try.

The music was instrumental and was very soothing for most people, I suppose. For me, it wasn't. I found my heart beating along with the beat of the music and was unable to get the sound of it out of my head. I could almost feel the notes bouncing up and down on the scale inside my body. I not only couldn't visualize the black velvet curtain that usually helped me to relax—white notes kept bouncing along like a bouncing ball—but I also couldn't find my mental hilltop or the swing. I almost could feel my muscles popping in time to the music.

I hesitated at first, not wanting to hurt her feelings, especially after she had brought the tape along to make me feel better. Then I remembered what I had learned about being assertive. I thanked her for her thoughtfulness, but said music wasn't working for me. She turned the tape off and I was able to switch into the relaxation mode almost at once.

You might find that experience strange. Others I've told it to say in surprise, "But I fall asleep to music on the clock radio." I'm sure they do, but I can't. That's why it's so important to take your time to discover what works best for you. The ability to relax at will is important for everyone, but especially so if you're trying to gain relief from IBS. It's certainly worth an investment of your time. This investment, unlike some of the financial ones you may have made lately, will pay off extremely well in the long run.

You really need to become a "You" consultant, and know as much about yourself as you can. You probably already check your body for the usual things—suspicious lumps, moles, pimples, gray hair, and added weight—so start inventorying your tension quotient as well.

How to find time to practice relaxation

You'll never find time to practice relaxation techniques; you have to make it. That is, you have to take it away from something else. It's like exercise, making love, and any other activity that's important in your life. If you don't consider it a priority, there won't be time for it.

There is time, of course. We all waste hours of precious time every day, nervously tapping our fingers on the desk or sales counter, jiggling coins in our pocket, biting fingernails, and pulling on or playing with our hair. These all are expressions of tension, moments that could be far better spent evoking a sense of tranquillity and deep relaxation.

Next time you're in the back of a cab caught in a traffic jam, take off your watch. If you're late for the next appointment, you're late. Adding stress to the moment certainly won't make you feel any better, nor will it get you there on time. Instead, lean back against the seat, close your eyes, and concentrate on your breathing. Visualize your relaxing spot or mentally focus on your special word or phrase. When

you finally arrive where you're going, you should feel much
better.

Some people prefer to take a relaxation break after they've
exercised; others, as soon as they awake in the morning. I
prefer taking time-out around four in the afternoon. I practice ten to fifteen minutes of deep relaxation, followed by
my latest craze, a cup of hot cinnamon tea. After my half-
hour break, I feel totally relaxed, energized, and ready for
almost anything.

Relaxation is not a cure

Although all these relaxation techniques can help you to
manage much of the stress in your life, they cannot eliminate it altogether, nor can they give you a cure for irritable
bowel syndrome. What they can do, however, is to teach
you how to minimize the *effect* of stress on your entire body,
especially, your digestive tract.

Most IBS sufferers admit that stress and emotional tension trigger their symptoms. If you have ever taken the time
to plot the course of your symptoms—from the first time
you recall ever having problems to the most recent episode—you may find a recurring pattern. If new situations,
holidays, or late hours tend to trigger your symptoms, spend
extra time practicing your relaxation techniques beforehand.
Let your detection diaries clue you in to the time of greatest
stress for you. Plan ahead for situational stress by scheduling more relaxation breaks.

Relaxation therapy is usually used in conjunction with
other methods to help control the symptoms of IBS. Most
experts feel that some form of stress management training
is a vital part of the treatment of irritable bowel syndrome.
Hypnosis has been used by a few researchers as a means to
induce relaxation. As stress is part of our lives, the trick is
not to avoid it, but rather, to learn to control its negative
effect on us.

A sample script for achieving deep relaxation

This is what I originally used when I practiced relaxation at home. It is what works for me, not what I specifically recommend for you.

If you work with a psychologist, psychiatrist, or other professional trained in the use of relaxation, he or she will probably give you written instructions specifically for your use. If not, you may have to discover what works best for you through a trial and error process.

I do believe, however, from talking to people who practice relaxation, that what you say is not as important as the fact that you have scheduled within your day a specific time to relax and to teach your body what relaxation feels like. As you've seen in this chapter, there are many ways to achieve this tranquil state. It's worth the effort to experience it.

When I begin to relax, my eyes are closed. I am relaxed. I slowly breathe in and out, in and out, feeling my body relax, feeling light, feeling as though I am floating. I breathe in and out. With my eyes closed, I see velvet, black, a black velvet curtain. I think, "Calm. I am calm.

"I am calm. My toes are warm. Warm toes. Relaxed. My feet are warm. Relaxed. I am calm. My ankles are warm. Heavy. Relaxed. I am calm.

"My legs are warm. Warm legs. Relaxed. I am calm. My knees are warm. Warm legs. Relaxed. Calm. I am calm. My thighs are warm. Warm thighs. Relaxed. Calm. I am calm.

"My hips are warm. Warm hips. Relaxed. Calm. I am calm. My waist is warm. Warm waist. Relaxed. Calm. I am calm. My chest is warm. Warm chest. Relaxed. Calm. I am calm.

"My fingers are warm. Warm fingers. Relaxed. Calm. I am calm. My wrists are warm. Warm wrists. Relaxed. Calm. I am calm. My arms are warm. Warm arms. Relaxed. Calm. I am calm.

"My shoulders are warm. Warm shoulders. Relaxed.

Calm. I am calm. My neck is warm. Warm neck. Relaxed. Calm. I am calm.

"My chin is warm. Warm chin. Relaxed. Calm. I am calm. My lips are warm. Warm lips. Relaxed. Calm. I am calm. My cheeks are warm. Warm cheeks. Relaxed. Calm. I am calm. My eyelids are warm. Warm eyelids. Relaxed. Calm. I am calm. My forehead is warm. Warm forehead. Relaxed. Calm. I am calm."

Then I continue to breathe in and out, and let myself float to my "spot," the swing. As the swing goes back, I inhale. As it goes forward, I exhale and think, "calm." When I'm ready to return to work, I count backward from five, open my eyes and feel refreshed.

That's it. Nothing magical or strange. It makes *me* relaxed. I hope it, or whatever you use for your own relaxation, helps you. If you adapt this or write your own, do let your physician or mental health professional see what you've written before you give it a try. He or she may have some most helpful additions or deletions.

After I have used the above to relax, I feel refreshed, warm, and comfortable. I feel like smiling. Best of all, I don't feel tense.

14

Learning Biofeedback

Biofeedback—also known as "operant" or "target" conditioning—is yet another technique that can be used to achieve relaxation and thereby gain some relief for those suffering from IBS spasms.

What is biofeedback?

Biofeedback is a therapy involving the use of electronic monitoring equipment that gives you instantaneous information on the state of your body's brain waves, heart rate, skin temperature, and muscle tension so that you can learn to change or control those functions and thereby reduce pain and stress. It's the mechanical version of the body's normal feedback systems, such as feeling your nose itch and "telling" your arm to scratch it, or feeling cold or frightened and shivering.

Through the marvels of modern machinery, biofeedback allows you to become aware of your body's internal signals and learn to regulate or at least begin to voluntarily control many of them. It's a relatively new science, only named by researchers in 1969.

How does biofeedback work?

Biofeedback training is usually administered by a psychologist or physician trained in the use of this type of monitoring device. The subject (the person on whom the biofeedback equipment is being used) sits comfortably in a chair or lies on a couch or padded table. Often, the lights are dimmed. Electrical terminals called "electrodes" are attached to different areas of the head and body. It is *not* painful as they're attached with a type of paste or tape. There is no sensation *from* the equipment to the subject since the electronic signals come from the body and are fed into the machine where they are transformed into visual or audio readings.

The level of the person's internal body activity is revealed continuously by aural or visual signals, such as a low beep or hum, a light, a number scale, or a picture. Eventually, after a period of practice, the subject will begin to see a relationship between what he or she is experiencing and what is being projected audiolly or visually. It doesn't mean that the person instantly will be able to control muscle tension and reduce stress. It does mean, however, that the individual will soon learn what the beginning sensations of tension and stress feel like and can quickly shift into relaxation techniques designed to prevent stress from taking hold.

What can it do?

Through biofeedback training, people have learned to lower their skin temperature, which helps eliminate migraine headaches. Others have learned to slow their heart rate, lower blood pressure, and in some cases minimize spasms in their intestinal tract.

Unlike progressive relaxation, in which you learn to detect your tension areas and then relax them, biofeedback works more quickly by instantly signaling you through sound, color, or other visual cues that you are tense. Once you learn to reduce the tension level cued electronically, you soon begin to recognize the sensations without the machinery and can reduce tension at will.

Although biofeedback fails to deal with the emotional components of IBS, it has been used successfully by some psychologists, physicians, and researchers to treat the stress that triggers discomforting symptoms of irritable bowel syndrome. Although researchers like Dr. William E. Whitehead have used biofeedback, both specifically targeted to relax the intestinal tract and generally to induce total body relaxation, Whitehead feels the latter technique seems to be more effective.

Researchers C. Madeline Mitchell, M.U.R.P., and Douglas A. Drossman, M.D., say that "specific biofeedback training using the patients' intracolonic motor activity as the basis for response, is still under investigation."[1] A preliminary study showed there was improvement in intestinal motility but there was not a corresponding change in symptoms.[2]

In general, biofeedback seems to be most effective with those who have strong motivation to be actively involved in handling their own treatment, to be participants rather than passive recipients. It is particularly helpful when the person is aware of his or her particular muscular tension and other physiological responses to stress. Biofeedback may enhance the response.[3] It also is often used in combination with other treatments, especially therapy designed to teach stress coping skills.

As with all of the other forms of treatment, biofeedback may work for some people and not others. At best, it is an aid, not a cure. It is more expensive than some of the other relaxation techniques as it employs the use of high-technology equipment, necessitates someone with experience to operate it, and usually requires your going to the doctor's office or a clinic to learn to use it. Once the technique is mastered, of course, you no longer are dependent on the electronic monitoring devices and can practice biofeedback alone at home.

Availability of biofeedback equipment and trained personnel may be a problem, depending on where you live. But biofeedback is an option and one that might be considered.

For more information on biofeedback and other relaxation therapies and a list of referrals in your area, contact your local hospital or send a stamped, self-addressed envelope to:

Biofeedback Society of America
10200 West 44th Avenue
Suite 304
Wheat Ridge, Colorado 80033

15

Exercising

Until very recently, the last time I really enjoyed exercise was when I was ten and played football with my male buddies in the backyard. Then I learned that "girls don't play sports," the dictum in my day when girls' basketball rules in my state only allowed females to run half court.

My college had physical education requirements, much to my dismay. I satisfied the requirement if not myself by taking fencing, although they had no left-handed protection jacket and I had to wear mine inside out, and folk dancing, a freshman course left until my senior year. Today I still suffer anxiety attacks when I hear a polka.

Why exercise?

Why exercise now, when no school requirements hang over your head? Why exercise, when just the thought of changing clothes is exhausting and works you into a sweat? Why? I guess it's because even if you don't enjoy doing it, you feel better *after* it is done. What's more, the gym teacher was right. It *is* good for you.

Regardless how far the ads tell us we have come, we're still not that far from our cave-dwelling ancestors. Our nervous system remains much the same. Early man (and woman) needed to be quickly prepared for what physiologist Walter B. Cannon termed the "fight or flight" response in order to survive. When faced with unexpected hostile beasts

147

or invading clans, digestion shut down, heart rate and blood pressure rose, and oxygen intake increased. Muscles tensed. Our ancestors were ready! And the active readiness state of their bodies was beneficial for existence in the world in which they lived.

Times change, of course. But our nervous system hasn't. Our bodies still react in the same way when we're bumped in the subway, cut off by a kid in the next lane, or told off by our boss. Unfortunately, we can't very well come out swinging or run away. Instead, the state of "readiness" hurts our bodies by creating unreleased tension, resulting in heart attacks, strokes, decreased immunity, and painful IBS.

The previous chapters have discussed ways in which we can use the mind to dilute our "readiness" state and promote relaxation. This chapter deals with ways in which physical activity can help achieve the same effect—while also helping us to lose weight, firm up, and look and feel better at the same time. As exercise improves your stamina, you get fatigued less easily, and fatigue, as you may remember, is one of the triggers of IBS symptoms for many people.

What type of exercise is "best"?

Fortunately, there is no "best" exercise to reduce stress. There is a wide variety, from aerobics, baseball and basketball, cycling and climbing, dancing, fencing, golf and gymnastics, hiking and handball, ice hockey, judo and jogging, and karate, to rowing and racketball, soccer, swimming and softball, tennis, volleyball, walking, and water skiing.

Some people try only one form of exercise and when they decide they really don't like that particular activity, they hang up their sweat suits forever. It needn't be. You just need to discover those forms of exercise that best suit you, your lifestyle, and your pocketbook. But do some thinking first so you don't sabotage your efforts. The idea is to *encourage* yourself to exercise, not to discourage yourself.

Before you run out to buy skis and cute skiing outfits, ask

yourself if you really like cold weather and heights and can afford to get to ski areas. Don't join a basketball group if you prefer to exercise alone. Everyone's different. Some people cherish the solitude of running, walking, or swimming laps and get their best ideas as they bounce along, while others look forward to exercise as a form of socializing.

How much are you able and willing to spend on exercise? While there's no need to go into debt for a particular form of exercise—there are too many others to choose from—you can figure in your budget that money spent for exercise will probably be money saved in doctor's bills. Most people who exercise regularly say it makes them feel better physically and mentally and that it acts like a tranquilizing shield, protecting them from the stress bullets being fired throughout their workday.

Can you pace yourself so you don't burn out or become compulsive about exercise? Unfortunately, many people throw themselves into whatever form of exercise they have selected with such fervor and obsessiveness that they end up negating any benefits because they have created *more* stress—both physical and emotional—through their competitiveness. You've probably seen them on the tennis court with eyes narrowed, facial muscles taut, ready to slam the ball down their opponent's throat at any moment. Or they ride the golf course range on their trusty carts, jamming tees into the ground with force that would detonate any grenade, and throwing clubs in frustration when they fail to perform. Aids to relaxation? Never!

While many people enjoy jogging, it, too, can become a harmful addiction. Many sports-medicine specialists see athletic addicts who continue to run on stress fractures, with tendinitis, with fever, and even with pneumonia. Some who also suffer from the eating disorder of anorexia obsessively run to burn off the few calories they have consumed.

Running, of course, does have positive results including stress reduction and muscle tone, but it should, as with most things, be done in moderation. You're not training for the Olympics. Irritable bowel sufferers who are prone to constipation will find that jogging does stimulate bowel movements. Vigorous runners, however, may suffer from diarrhea.

Grandfather's "daily constitutional"—walking briskly—still holds its own as a safe, beneficial, and lifelong form of exercise. While some of us are "closet walkers," clocking our miles in privacy on the treadmill while watching soaps, videos, or daily news reports, most walkers seem to prefer the out-of-doors—seeing people, enjoying the changing seasons, and breathing fresh air, or what passes for it in most of our cities.

Swimming is another exercise that reduces stress and conditions the body without putting too much strain on the joints. It's especially good for those with arthritis or who need the buoyancy of the water, such as those who have bad knees. You can start slowly and compete with yourself, adding laps as you see fit. Never swim alone. Even expert swimmers have been known to suffer serious cramps.

Although some people keep records of their laps, miles run, sets played, etc., I suggest restraint. Those who tend to be competitive (most IBS sufferers are) sometimes become driven to beat their friend's time, overexerting themselves and creating serious additional stress. If you must log in your exercise prowess for "bragging rights," keep track only of the amount of time you spent, not how much distance you covered or how fast you were. In the beginning, you may walk only a short distance in your twenty to forty minutes. As you relax and get more in shape, you'll probably pick up speed and cover more distance in that same time period.

If you think you'd like a type of exercise requiring expensive equipment, such as cross-country skiing, treadmill, or bike-racing, see if you can borrow or rent the equipment first. Don't assume you'll use it because it cost a lot of money. If all the unused stationary bikes in America were laid end to end, I bet they'd reach from California to North Carolina!

Although not an aerobic form of exercise, many physicians suggest sit-ups and leg-lifts for IBS sufferers. These and other exercises specifically designed to tone and firm up stomach muscles are important, as strong stomach muscles are better able to maintain pressure on the walls of the intestine. This helps control constipation problems.

When is there time for exercise?

Never! You'll have to *make* time for exercise. It may mean getting up a little earlier than usual or going to the gym during lunch hour. Some people with flexible working hours leave the office in time to get their walking or running in before dark. Cut an hour from your television viewing and use that for exercise—or if you can't bear the thought of missing a single show, put an exercise bike, rowing machine, or cross-country ski machine in front of the set. If the cost of this type of equipment is prohibitive, buy a jump rope or run in place. Gotcha! There's really no excuse for not exercising.

Make sure you find the time of day that is best for you. If you're a night person, you may find it hard to discipline yourself to rise at dawn for exercise. Before dinner might be a better "fit." An added advantage of exercising at the end of the day is that it helps ease the tension collected throughout the day, especially if it's been "one of those days." Whenever you schedule your workout, try to look forward to doing it, or at least to having done it. Don't lose sight of the fact that exercise should be enjoyed. Your purpose is to feel better by reducing stress, not to become tense with resentment and frustration.

Don't try to get all your exercise done on the weekends. Hospital emergency rooms are filled with "weekend jocks" who are sedentary all week and then try to work out all the kinks over the weekend. Instead, they pull muscles, overwork their bodies, and trigger excess stress.

It's much more beneficial to get in some type of exercise at least three times during the week for twenty to forty minutes. Park a distance from your place of work or shopping and walk there; head for the gym during lunch hour or go for a leisurely bike ride. You'll have more energy for the rest of the day and feel less pressured.

If you prefer out-of-doors exercise, have a rainy day plan as well so you don't use bad weather as an excuse to skip exercise. It's easy to procrastinate. You can always think of a good reason to put it off. Of course, the best reason to make time for exercise is *you*.

Vary your exercise

There are many ways of exercising—alone, in groups such as aerobic or dance classes, or in teams, either organized like a softball or soccer league or a friendly pick-up basketball game. To keep from becoming bored, vary your form of exercise. If you do calisthenics alone at home in front of the mirror or the television, for example, also schedule some of your exercise time to play tennis or softball with friends. Many people feel that it's easiest to keep up a regular workout routine when they have a partner depending on them to show up.

Exercise should be fun

The important thing to remember when you're using exercise to reduce stress is that it should be *FUN*. Often we forget that. We're working so hard to play well that we forget to play.

We need to try to recapture some of the fun of childhood, when we ran around playing cops and robbers, or cowboys, or just ran. We didn't think about exercise when we hopped on our bike and rode to a friend's house or when we played dodge ball or tag. We just played, having fun and letting our bodies expend energy that had been bottled up inside during school hours.

Remember how the wind and snow burned your cheeks as you ran and then belly-flopped on your sled when you were a kid? How you felt warm and exhilarated after lapping your big brother in the pool? How relaxed and sleepy you were after pedaling uphill to the lake? Remember these sensations. You had exercised, only you didn't know you were supposed to call it that. You were having fun; you also weren't having any stress.

Additional benefits

Exercise seems almost like a magic elixir that promises us the world. While it can't quite deliver that, regular exercise does put the twinkle back in our eye. Because our tension level is lowered through exercise, we feel better physically and mentally and feel better about ourselves as well.

We look better, too. Regular exercise boosts the metabolism, so we burn up calories faster. We not only lose weight, but fat turns to muscle so we look more fit. Joint flexibility is increased as well.

There tends to be a ripple effect. People who begin to exercise regularly usually become more conscious of their other health habits. Many former smokers said that, after years of trying every "stop smoking" program available, the experience that made them able to give it up was the "high" they received through exercise.

"I felt it was stupid to feel so good running and then poison my system by smoking," said one former smoker. "Running seemed more satisfying by that point and I was able to quit at last."

Heart specialists usually recommend regular brisk walking, running, swimming, or cycling to lower the dangers of coronary heart disease.

The list goes on. There's really no good reason why you shouldn't start a regular exercise program. What are you waiting for?

Always check with your doctor first

It's always a good idea to get a physical checkup from your doctor before you begin any exercise program.

16

Dining Gracefully

My grandmother used to say, "Animals eat; people dine." She obviously lived before the days of drive-in restaurants, stand-up restaurant bars, and eating on the run. But, as with many of our grandparents' sayings, hers made a great deal of sense.

How do you eat?

Study your detection diaries to see if your IBS symptoms often center around mealtimes or snacks. If you begin to see a pattern, your problem may not be as much *what* you are eating, but *how* you are eating it.

Think about your eating habits. Do you:

- eat standing up?
- swallow without chewing thoroughly?
- chew with your mouth open?
- wash your food down with water or other beverages?
- eat while you're working at your desk?
- eat while you talk on the phone?
- jump up and down from the table during your meal?

If you answer yes to any of these, you're adding more to your diet than calories. You're increasing your stress level and forcing your already uneasy intestinal tract to work even harder.

As described in Chapter 2, your digestive tract goes to work on food as soon as it hits the mouth. It's actually working even before that, especially when your mouth begins to water as you sniff and recognize the unmistakable aroma of freshly baked bread, roast turkey, or whatever food scents appeal to you.

When you add mealtime tension, air swallowed with food, or poorly chewed food to your intestine's chore, you can expect trouble. But by changing some of your poor mealtime habits to more positive ones, you can begin to reduce much of the tension you experience while you eat, as well as the discomfort that follows.

Set the mood

Picture a romantic dinner with someone you love. The table is in a quiet nook, away from the clatter of dishes, ringing telephones, and screaming kids. You and your special person sit across from each other, smiling over the flickering candles. The table is set with a beautiful cloth, fine china, and sparkling silverware. Soft music plays in the background.

Sounds great, doesn't it? But for many, dinner is in the kitchen with the television blaring, serving us murders and other violence either as news or regular programming. The telephone is ringing, the kids are fighting, and everyone seems to be hopping up and down like players in a musical farce. A family I know had an extra long cord attached to their phone so they could talk on the phone as they ate dinner. Relaxing fare? Hardly.

While most of us can't very well dine out every night, we can learn to dine graciously in our own homes. We can learn—and teach our children at the same time—how to treat the most important company we'll ever entertain: ourselves and our families.

Many people have "good" dishes which they never use. They're saving them. What for? For their kids to inherit, I guess. But wouldn't it be a greater gift to give the children memories of relaxing family dinners, seated around the prettiest table possible, using the good china? Add a few candles, soft music on the stereo or radio, and pleasant conversation. Now *that's* dining! It doesn't matter if you're eating pheasant under glass or hamburger in the bun. If the mood is one of calmness and the pace is leisurely, you're dining.

Don't let the fact that your children are young keep you on the dinner dash circuit. Start small. Set aside one night a week for leisurely dining. Let the children help set the table, plan a centerpiece, and even prepare some of the meal. Most youngsters enjoy working in the kitchen and soon develop their own culinary specialties. Also, when they've helped cook dinner, they're more willing to sample new foods.

Encourage everyone to dress up just a little that night to make it more special. You may be surprised to find that even your "picky" eaters eat a little better when the mood is calmer. Your intestinal tract may behave a little better as well.

If you do have a young family, plan another special dinner for just you and your spouse. Either feed the children early so the two of you can eat later when things are quieter, or do as I did when I had four toddlers in the house. My husband and I had a standing Wednesday night date. The babysitter was prebooked so we had no reason to procrastinate. On the contrary. We looked forward to our relaxing Wednesday night dinner for two. Because it was midweek, it also tended to slow us down if our pace had become a little too frantic, which it usually had.

How to dine alone

To me, mealtime is also a social event. The conversation served up is as important as what's on my plate, and often even more so. For that reason, I always hated to eat alone. When I did, I was likely to eat cereal, a pint of ice cream, or a bowl of popcorn. A book or magazine was my companion and, caught up in the pages, I usually was oblivious to what I was eating. My detection diaries revealed that I often suffered more discomfort from IBS symptoms after I dined alone.

Then I thought about my late mother-in-law. She was a very dear lady and, by the time I married her youngest son, she was a widow and lived alone. Yet each night for dinner, she set her table in the dining room with a linen placemat, her best china, and silverware. Despite her small appetite, she always fixed meat or chicken, a potato, a vegetable, and salad. When she made Jell-O, she served it in a special little silver bowl she had received for a wedding gift and which had the date inscribed on the bottom.

I remember asking her why she went through such a bother when it was only for herself.

"Why not?" she answered, in the Jewish tradition of answering a question with another question. "Aren't I important to myself? Who should I save it for? I enjoy being nice to me."

Now I have her little silver bowl and I, too, pour Jell-O into it to cool. We still eat dinner in our dining room, as we always have, even when the children were small, and continue to use our best dishes and silver even though we're "just" family. Although conversation is somewhat more elevated than when they were younger and it consisted mostly of "Mother, tell him not to look at me," and "She kicked me first," it is hardly stuff that Henry Kissinger or William Buckley would boast of. But it usually is pleasant and relaxed.

When I eat alone, I now try to think of Mama, my mother-in-law, and make mealtime special for me. I put on a new tape or CD, get out a placemat, and ban stress and tension from my table. My mind wanders. I'm relaxed. Alone with my thoughts, I have discovered that dinner for one, although not my first choice, can be an enjoyable experience.

Slow down

Did your mother tell you to slow down and not gobble your dinner? Mine did. I wanted to get through and go back outside to play until it got dark.

I later learned the hard way that eating too rapidly may trigger IBS symptoms. You not only gulp down large quantities of air, which can cause gas and bloating, but you also create extra tension in the digestive system. While I don't suggest chewing your food twenty times before swallowing, I personally found that making an effort to eat more slowly helped reduce my symptoms.

If you find that you're usually through eating long before anyone else, try putting your fork down between bites and really listening to what the other person is saying. You'll feel more relaxed, probably enjoy the meal more now that you're taking the time to smell and taste it, and be less uncomfortable when you're through.

If you're on a tight schedule and really rushed for time, eat less and eat lightly. An apple or banana and cheese-on-whole-wheat-bread sandwich eaten leisurely, with time for a brief stroll afterward, will relax you more than trying to hurriedly cram a hamburger, fries, and a milk shake or coffee into an already tense digestive tract.

When you expect a particularly stressful or rushed day, plan ahead for lunchtime. Leave early so you won't have to stand in line or gulp your meal when you do get a table. If you can't leave early, bring a light bag lunch so you can dine gracefully. Eating should leave you refreshed and relaxed, not taxed.

By planning ahead for meals, especially during times of stress, you also give yourself ''time out'' to consider what would be best for you to eat. That way you're less likely to grab the first thing you see, which invariably is something containing either too much fat or too much sugar. Both can trigger IBS symptoms.

Don't overeat

When six IBS sufferers compared their detection diaries recently, they discovered that each of them had experienced severe pain, gas, and discomfort during the holidays. All admitted to feeling more stress during these family-oriented events, but in addition, all said they had overeaten.

"I really felt stuffed at Thanksgiving," said one. "I was full before dessert, but ate the pumpkin pie anyway. My mother makes great pumpkin pie. I couldn't hurt her feelings."

In addition to rereading Chapter 9 on assertiveness (how to tell Mom you love her, even though you don't want any of her pumpkin pie just now), this person also needed to think about what she was doing to her already overstressed digestive system. Since the amount of hormones released when you eat increases with the increasing size of your meal, overeating dumps more symptom-triggering chemicals into your intestinal tract. Was she sure that was what she wanted to do?

It's far better to eat smaller, more frequent meals than to overtax your intestinal tract when it's already feeling tension. Even those without irritable bowel syndrome feel uncomfortable when they overeat. For IBS sufferers, it's almost one of life's sure things.

The idea's not new. Wise men have been teaching moderation in all things over the centuries. The seventeenth-century English poet Robert Herrick (who also penned the line, "Gather ye Rosebuds while ye may") wrote:

> Go to your banquet, then, but use delight,
> So as to rise still with an appetite.

It's often not what you eat

When you have IBS, it's easy to blame all your pain and discomfort on food—what you eat. But by reducing your stress level through the techniques described in this and previous chapters, you should be able to come to the table more relaxed and be able to enjoy the entire experience of dining—the taste of good food, the ambience, the companionship of friends and family, and interesting conversation.

Adding Fiber

"Eat more fiber."

It sounds so easy, doesn't it? Deceptively so. It fails to address some important questions, such as: What is fiber? Where do you get it? How much is enough? Is fiber good for everyone?

Before the 1970s, people with irritable bowel syndrome, as well as those with many other bowel disorders, were usually put on bland diets and told to avoid roughage in their diets.

Since the mid-1970s, however, thanks to the work of two British researchers and physicians, Drs. Denis Burkitt and Hubert Trowell, "fiber" has been the buzzword. The media have picked it up and heralded fiber as the salvation of America, if not the entire civilized world. Ironically, according to Dr. Chesley Hines, Jr., of Tulane University School of Medicine and Louisiana State University School of Medicine, "The average daily consumption of dietary fiber in the United States is less than 25 grams a day whereas dietary fiber intake in less developed countries may be as high as 60 to 90 grams a day."[1] The National Cancer Institute recommends that we eat foods that provide 25 to 35 grams of fiber per day (28 grams = 1 ounce). For many people this means their daily intake of fiber should be doubled.

What is fiber?

So less developed countries eat more fiber than most Americans do. So what? What is fiber, anyway?

Fiber is not a magical substance, nor a modern-day cure-all. Known also as "bulk" or "roughage," fiber is a collective term for the bits of plant material that cannot be digested no matter how hard the juices in the small intestine try. Remember what you read in Chapter 2? Digestion takes place in the small intestine. What cannot be digested there passes into the colon where the water portion is absorbed and the remainder is expelled as feces through the rectum.

Fiber helps to regulate bowel function by aiding in the formation of soft, smooth, easy-to-pass stools and by shortening intestinal transit time. It has the ability to absorb the excess water that causes loose stools and at the same time relieves constipation by adding the necessary bulk to stimulate a bowel movement.

Actually, there are two types of fiber: soluble and insoluble. Soluble fiber forms gels in water and is found in beans, some fruits, vegetables, oats, and barley. According to recent research, soluble fiber tends to help lower blood cholesterol levels and regulate the body's use of glucose.

Insoluble fiber doesn't dissolve in water and has as its main component cellulose. It's found in wheat bran, whole grains, and many vegetables. Insoluble fiber retains water in the gastrointestinal tract, thus increasing bulk, softening the stools, hastening transit time, and thus aiding in elimination.

You needn't worry about which fiber is which, however, if you consult with your physician or a nutritionist or registered dietitian and learn what foods make up a high-fiber diet. You can find the names of registered dietitians in your area by contacting your physician, local hospitals, or your state Dietetic Association. You'll find more information on how to find a qualified nutritionist or registered dietitian in Chapter 18.

Where can you get fiber?

Fiber is found naturally, but in varying degrees, in a number of food products, including:

Vegetables

- broccoli
- cabbage
- brussels sprouts
- corn
- carrots
- beets
- celery
- cauliflower
- potatoes (baked in their skins and eaten with the skin)

Fruits

- prunes
- raisins
- strawberries
- oranges
- peaches
- apricots
- blackberries
- pears
- bananas
- cantaloupes
- apples (Remember what grandma said about "An apple a day"? It seems she was right, especially when you eat the peel as well. Apples contain pectin fiber, which traps excess fat and moves it quickly through the digestive system before the body can absorb it.)

Additional Sources

- nuts
- popcorn
- lentils
- brown rice
- peas
- kidney beans
- dark breads (such as whole-wheat and pumpernickel)
- whole meal crackers (We call them graham crackers and the English call them digestives.)
- cereals (Especially those containing bran, wheat, and oats. Avoid those with sugar, as they contain too many empty calories and can create extra gas.)

When you're shopping for bread, take a few moments to read the label. The highest fiber content is in the bread with the *least* processing. If the first ingredient on the label is "100% whole meal flour," "cracked wheat," "stone-ground wheat," "sprouted wheat," "wheat bran," "whole rye flour," "oat bran," or "oatmeal," there is a higher fiber content than if the first ingredient is enriched wheat flour.

Eating bran—especially unprocessed bran or "miller's bran," which can be purchased in health food stores or groceries—is an easy way to increase your fiber intake. If you have a choice between coarse or fine flakes, select the former as they're more effective. As unprocessed bran tends to taste like I imagine sawdust would taste, you'll probably want to add it to your cereal or fruit salad, mix it with yogurt, or sprinkle it on a sandwich or on your cottage cheese. Add bran to whole meal flour and bake your own bran bread. Oat bran, which is now available in most groceries and health food stores, is also a good source of fiber and, like wheat bran, makes good muffins—especially when you add a handful of raisins.

Fiber by itself provides no nutrition and contains almost no calories. Fiber-rich foods also require more chewing, so you feel satisfied more quickly. That's one of the reasons it's better to eat an apple whole than to drink apple juice. Another reason is that, according to the United States Department of Agriculture, three-quarters of a cup of apple juice contains only 0.2 grams of fiber, whereas a whole apple, with its peel, contains 3.6 grams of fiber.

In addition, these fiber-rich foods provide bulk so you tend to eat less of high-calorie foods. Isn't it a nice plus to know that along with helping you regulate your bowels, extra fiber in your diet can also help you lose pounds or maintain your weight?

Use high-fiber foods for snacks, too. You can choose among sesame bread sticks, Fig Newtons, date or prune bars, date or prune bread, and oatmeal cookies with raisins. They're not only good between-meal treats that are good for you, they also add fiber, which helps you feel full.

There are certain plant seeds called "psyllium," used
to make bulking agents known as "psyllium hydrophilic
mucilloid," which can also add fiber to your diet. Products like Metamucil and Effer-Syllium contain psyllium
and are a convenient way to slowly increase the fiber in
your diet. They are particularly effective for those with
IBS who suffer primarily from constipation, although
many with diarrhea as their main complaint also get relief. Do *not* confuse these products with chemical laxative
preparations. These are natural products and do not have
serious side effects. Most of them come in powder form
and are mixed with water, fruit juices, or even iced
tea.

Increase your fluid intake

It's important to increase your consumption of liquids—
preferably water—when you increase the amount of fiber in
your diet. Failure to drink enough fluids can cause constipation or make existing conditions more severe. Most physicians suggest drinking six to eight eight-ounce glasses of
water daily.

If you're not much of a water drinker, give yourself specific reminders. I put eight water glasses out on the kitchen
counter each morning on a special tray. By evening, I should
have used them all. My sister put eight pennies on her win-
dowsill. As she drank a glass of water, she'd transfer a penny
into an egg cup. Use a chart, a pitcher on your office desk,
or whatever it takes to remind you, but do drink enough
water.

How much is enough?

You may think you already get enough fiber in your diet,
but chances are you don't. Most Americans eat only about
15 to 20 grams of dietary fiber each day. Although doctors
tend to vary in their opinion of how much we *should* be
eating, most of them do agree that it should be in the 25 to
35 gram range. With all the highly processed foods in the

American diet, it takes some planning to eat that much fiber. It's hard to eat it all in food alone.

If you're adding unprocessed bran to your food, start slowly, with about one or two heaping tablespoons on your cereal or salad. Increase the dosage slowly. There is no one amount that's right for everyone. Each person is an individual and one person may need less or more bran than another. It really becomes a trial and error situation until you find the amount that helps you have a bowel movement without straining but isn't so much that you have additional cramping and diarrhea.

Neither bran nor bulking agents should be considered a one-dose, fast-acting treatment for IBS. Go slowly. If you overdo it, trying to get relief in one day by cramming too much additional fiber into your intestine in too short a time, you'll suffer extreme discomfort.

Is fiber good for everyone?

There is some disagreement among researchers as to the benefits of fiber for all IBS patients. A recent study by P.A. Cann and Associates found that although fiber did help those IBS patients with constipation, it had little effect on those who suffered primarily from diarrhea.[2]

Although there is still considerable disagreement over the number of IBS patients with food intolerance—British researchers V. Alun Jones and J.O. Hunter suggest that "approximately 70 percent of those with abdominal pain and diarrhoea [sic] may be successfully managed by diet"[3]—it is obvious that anyone with a true allergy to wheat, one of the most common offending foods, would not improve on a diet high in wheat bran.

Be aware that almost everyone who greatly increases bran in his or her diet does experience some additional gas and bloating as the bacteria in the gut react to the fiber. But, according to Dr. Marvin M. Schuster, "this side effect disappears in 85 percent of patients after three weeks. Fifteen percent find it intolerable and have to discontinue bran."[4] If you are having troublesome side effects from the added bran, always discuss them with your physician before giving up on the additional fiber. You may have taken too much of the bran in your enthusiasm or you may need to be switched to one of the psyllium-seed preparations, such as Metamucil, which is mixed with water or fruit juice.

These bulking agents tend to work well for IBS sufferers with alternating diarrhea and constipation because they both absorb the excess water in the stool and soften the stool so it passes through the colon and into the rectum more easily. These products should be taken at mealtimes so they can mix with the stool as it is formed. Dr. Marvin M. Schuster adds, ''Because of taste factors and because some swelling of the psyllium seeds takes place in the stomach, there may be some appetite suppression if administered before meals. Therefore these agents should be taken by obese people before meals and by thin people after meals.''

Do *not* use chemical laxatives as a substitute for additional fiber in your diet. They quickly become habit forming, are too harsh for an intestinal tract already plagued with motility problems, and end up doing you more harm than good.

Suggested recipes to add fiber to your diet

Oat Bran Muffins

(This is an adaptation of the recipe on the box of Mother's Oat Bran. It makes a dozen muffins, which can be stored in a plastic bag in the refrigerator and then heated individually in the microwave or oven before eating.)

2½ cups oat bran cereal, uncooked
½ cup raisins
2 tsp. baking powder
¾ cup skim milk
scant ⅓ cup honey

2 eggs, beaten
2 Tbsp. vegetable oil

Heat oven to 425 degrees. Line muffin tin with paper baking
cups. Mix all ingredients in large bowl until dry ingredients
are moistened. Fill muffin cups evenly. (Should take no more
than 5 minutes to this point.) Bake 15 to 17 minutes. Muffins will not brown.

Hinks' Whole Meal Bread
Preheat oven to 375 degrees. Your actual working time is
only 25 minutes. The remainder of the time, dough is ris-
ing.

4 Tbsp. lukewarm water	**1 pkg. dry yeast**
2 cups lukewarm water	**2/3 cup powdered skim milk**
1 tsp. salt	**2 Tbsp. vegetable oil**
2 Tbsp. molasses	**2 Tbsp. honey**
4 2/3 cups 100% wheat flour	

Dissolve yeast in 4 Tbsp. lukewarm water and set aside.
Dissolve skim milk in 2 cups of lukewarm water in a big
bowl. Add salt, oil, molasses, and honey. Stir. Add dis-
solved yeast. Add wheat flour to mixture. Stir, cover with
clean dish towel, and set in warm place for one hour.

Grease and flour two loaf pans. Flour wooden board or
counter top. Knead dough for 10 minutes. Add flour if necessary to keep it from sticking. Knead additional 10 minutes.

Divide in two halves. Press into loaf pans. Cover with
cloth. Let dough rise one hour more.

Put pans on upper shelf of oven. On lower shelf, put pan
of hot water directly under the loaf pans.

Bake 50 minutes. Turn out on cooling rack. Enjoy!

For additional high-fiber recipes, plus a list of a variety
of foods along with their dietary fiber content, write for your

free copy of "Good News Booklet." Send your name and address to:

Good News Booklet
Kellogg Company, Dept. E-8
One Kellogg Square
Battle Creek, MI 49016-3599

═══ 18 ═══

Reviewing Your Eating Habits

One of the greatest difficulties doctors face in treating irritable bowel syndrome is in trying to pinpoint the particular triggers, especially when the symptoms themselves create additional stress. That makes your detection diaries (discussed in Chapter 7) all the more important. It's your opportunity to help your physician help you.

Don't jump to conclusions

When I interviewed Dr. Douglas Drossman, a specialist in dealing with IBS, he had this bit of advice he particularly wanted me to pass along.

"Warn your readers against being too quick to eliminate particular kinds of food from their diet," he said. "Often an IBS patient eats something, then the symptoms worsen, so the person decides it must be related to that food and avoids it entirely. Before too long, many foods are added to the 'can't eat' list and the person's diet is totally constricted."

Not only do some people create poorly balanced diets for themselves unnecessarily, they also make mealtimes more stressful for themselves as they worry about what they can and cannot eat. The added stress works against them, of course, usually triggering additional symptoms. The irony is that by restricting their diets so severely, they end up feeling worse, not better.

Slow down

That's not to say it isn't important to be aware of what you're eating. But as your detection diaries show, it's also important to become aware of your physical and psychological environment while you are eating as well as before and afterward.

As discussed in earlier chapters, many IBS sufferers report having pain, bloating, and diarrhea shortly after eating any meal, but particularly breakfast, regardless of what they've eaten. The act of eating triggers the abnormal contractions in the colon. In addition, however, many admit that their detection diaries noted that breakfast often was the "meal on the run." Trying to get everyone up, dressed, fed, and out the door to school and work shot their stress level up off the scale.

"By the time I get to work," sighed a thirty-five-year-old teacher, "I feel as though I swallowed a cannonball whole. I've tried skipping breakfast altogether, but I have as much, if not more, pain that way."

Try to slow things down in the morning, even if it means setting everyone's alarm fifteen minutes earlier. Set the table and put the cereal boxes, bowls, and juice glasses out on the counter. Save reading the paper for later. Put soothing music on the radio or stereo. Make a conscious attempt to move more slowly. Get up thirty minutes earlier and practice your relaxation techniques. Use your creativity to discover ways in which to switch to a more leisurely pace in the morning.

Eat more slowly

When you slow your eating, you chew your food better and swallow less air. Look around for clues. If you're always the first one finished, you're probably eating too quickly. Try putting your spoon or fork down between mouthfuls, cutting your food into smaller pieces, or pausing to really listen to what others are saying.

Don't speak with your mouth full. There is really very

little that must be said so urgently that you can't wait to carefully chew and swallow what's in your mouth. You also will be less likely to choke that way. Sharing a table with someone who talks with food in his or her mouth is an unappetizing sight. It can present awkward moments, as well. Recently, I sat next to someone who began talking before chewing what was in his mouth. He was a rather forceful fellow and accidentally spit part of his lunch onto my plate. It was an embarrassing moment for everyone.

Regulate your mealtimes

Check your detection diaries for the times your symptoms bother you the most. They may appear after irregular mealtimes. Eating at odd hours puts additional stress on a digestive tract that's already oversensitive. Try to eat your meals at the same time each day, especially on the weekends and during emotionally filled holidays.

When I first began keeping a detection diary, I discovered that many of my most uncomfortable days were during the weekends. I often tried to sleep late on Saturday and Sunday, thus missing breakfast and substituting brunch. As brunch usually was a restaurant or hotel buffet, I tended to eat more than usual. No wonder I felt bloated and uncomfortable the rest of the day. We also didn't eat dinner on weekends until late. My entire eating schedule was out of sync with the rest of the week. Once I began to keep fairly regular mealtime hours throughout the week, I had fewer problems with IBS symptoms.

Avoid fatty foods

That generally seems to be good advice for everyone, but it's especially so for IBS sufferers. Most people with irritable bowel syndrome tend to have more troublesome symptoms after eating fatty foods, including those which are greasy or fried. It's not surprising, as fat is the major dietary stimulant of the gastrocolic response.[1] The hormonal system releases chemicals to help digest the fat and they, particularly cholecystokinin (known as CCK), trigger additional abnormal movement in the colon.

Get help if you need it

Don't try to figure out your own nutritional requirements. If you have any doubts, ask your physician or local hospital for the name of a registered dietitian or qualified nutritionist. You also can contact your state American Dietetic Association or write to the national headquarters at 208 South LaSalle Street, Suite 1100, Chicago, IL 60604. In addition, there are specific physicians and clinicians who have received specialized training in nutrition. You can get the names of those in your area by sending a stamped, self-addressed envelope to the American Board of Nutrition, 9650 Rockville Pike, Bethesda, MD 20814.

These people are trained professionals who can help you analyze your detection diaries and advise you on how to avoid problem foods, add fiber, and decrease fat while still enjoying a balanced diet. They can also scrutinize your detection diaries for clues to situational stress that centers on eating habits and patterns.

Use care in selecting your nutritionist. Eating is a highly emotional issue and you need to be sure that you are comfortable with whomever you've selected. Once you've selected a nutritionist, be totally honest with him or her. Don't say what you think he or she wants to hear. The nutritionist's purpose is to help you feel better, not judge you.

Many people claim to be nutritionists when they actually have very little background or knowledge. Only a handful of states require nutritionists to be licensed, so don't hesitate to check a person's credentials or ask for references before letting someone handle your dietary planning. Your well-being may depend upon it.

Any food can be a problem for someone

Use your detection diaries to see what foods affect you, rather than relying on well-meaning advice from friends and family. Triggering foods vary widely. Almost any food can be a trigger for someone. The most common foods, however, are dairy products, citrus fruits, grains (such as wheat or corn), coffee and tea, cabbage, legumes, and food additives.

Women may be fooled into thinking they have problems with certain foods when the reaction coincides with their menstrual period. As many women suffer from constipation shortly before their period begins and diarrhea during and afterward, it's a good idea to mark those dates on the detection diaries.

Watch what you mix

Many IBS sufferers have a list of foods they *know* cause upsets—fatty foods like duck, fried chicken, some red meats, and whipped cream—but they often forget the foods they combine regularly, such as cereal with milk, bread with butter, or coffee with cream. Pastry also contains a high proportion of fat. Because we eat these combinations almost every day, they don't seem to "count." That's why it's important to record everything you eat on your detection diaries. They help you to remember the obvious.

See what you omit

Sometimes it's what you *don't* eat that creates problems. Since trying to lose weight for the last many years seems to have become a way of life for me, I often eat salads for lunch. In the past, I would skip breakfast, go out for lunch, and virtuously order a salad. Many times, even before the meal was finished, I was doubled up with pain.

When I began to keep detection diaries, I saw the pattern. Salads were no problem when I had eaten breakfast or when I ordered bread with the salad. It wasn't the salad, as such, that was creating my symptoms, but the fact that my stomach was empty when I began eating it.

Now I eat three meals a day. When I order salad for lunch, I order whole wheat toast with it. The carbohydrate from the bread seems to protect me.

Your personal intestinal body system may react in different ways to what you are omitting from your diet. Check your detection diaries to see if you can determine such a pattern.

Put pleasure on your plate

Eating is one of life's necessities, but it should be one that gives pleasure as well. While eating often does trigger discomfort for those of us with IBS, it also can be made more enjoyable by focusing on the senses rather than symptoms, sharing mealtime with interesting company, and taking time to savor the food. (Chapter 16 treats this subject in more detail.)

176 GUTSFROM IBS

19

Assessing Your Need For Medication

Sometimes everything you try isn't enough. Despite adding more fiber to your diet, regardless of the careful attention you pay to your detection diaries, no matter how much you try to relax and learn to handle stress, you still suffer from the pain and discomfort of IBS symptoms.

You haven't failed! It isn't all in your mind. It just means that you need to get back with your physician and discuss different types of medication to tide you over the rough spots. Remember, however, that irritable bowel syndrome is a chronic disorder. Don't expect a cure and don't get angry or frustrated with your doctor if he or she can't make all your discomfort go away. The idea is to titrate a dosage to give you relief, not to overmedicate you. While you don't need to be "macho" and suffer unnecessarily, it's always a good rule to try to use as little medication as possible.

Fiber first

Fortunately, there are a number of treatments for IBS, including dietary changes, exercise, and stress management, as well as drug therapy.

"Although the treatment for IBS must always be individualized," said Dr. Douglas A. Drossman, "my first line of treatment for all IBS patients is to increase fiber intake to about 15 to 20 grams a day."[1]

There are additional avenues of treatment for IBS including life-style and behavioral treatments (see Chapters 8 through 18) such as relaxation training, exercise programs, and psychological counseling, which may work by helping the person to understand and better adapt to the daily stresses in life that may aggravate the symptoms.

In addition, there are many drug therapies available, including anticholinergic prescription agents and other antispasmodics for pain, antidepressants for the depression that often comes with IBS, antidiarrheal drugs for diarrhea, bran and commercial bulking agents for constipation, and other drugs and preparations as required by the individual needs of the person. While physicians disagree as to the overall effectiveness of medications in the treatment of irritable bowel syndrome, most agree that short-term use when discomfort is at its peak can be useful.

Anticholinergics

Much of the pain felt by those suffering from IBS comes from cramps triggered by abnormal motor activity in the colon. Anticholinergics, also known as "antispasmodics," are a specific type of drug, such as Bentyl or Pro-Banthīne, that temporarily blocks nerve impulses to the muscles in the gut, thus reducing these painful spasms in the colon. This type of medication is often prescribed for use in those patients who suffer a great deal of pain and constipation.

Peppermint oil

Oil from the peppermint plant is often given in capsule form to people suffering from irritable bowel syndrome, especially in Europe.[2] The peppermint oil, coated and in capsule form to prevent its being absorbed before reaching the colon, inhibits gastrointestinal smooth muscle activity, thus reducing both gas and pain. Peppermint oil coated capsules are available at many health food stores and seem to have few side effects. However, as with all medications, peppermint oil should only be taken under a physician's guidance to be sure of getting the proper dosage.

Antidiarrheal agents

Antidiarrheal agents are drugs such as Lomotil or Imodium that have the ability to oppose or counteract diarrhea. Nonprescription antidiarrheal medications include Kaopectate and Pepto-Bismol. They relieve the sense of urgency by slowing down the colon's contractions and help to provide more solid stools. Their dosage must be carefully titrated to give the greatest effect without causing constipation.

Antidepressants

These drugs, such as Elavil, help some people to control the depressive feelings that are not uncommon with irritable bowel syndrome. Your doctor will determine whether or not your symptoms require an antidepressant and will take into consideration the effect any medication will have on bowel symptoms before prescribing for you.

Bulking agents

While some patients prefer to add fiber-rich foods to their diet or to increase bran, others find it easier to supplement their diet with commercial preparations of psyllium hydrophilic mucilloid. This is a natural therapeutic bulking agent and is *not* to be confused with chemical laxatives, which can become habit-forming and have unpleasant side effects.

The advantage of using these natural fiber products, such as Metamucil, is that the patient often finds them more convenient to use than adding additional fiber to the diet (and thus is more likely to be consistent in usage) and can easily increase or decrease the dosage until the desired response is obtained.

Understand your medications

It's not enough to ask your physician for medication to give you some relief from the discomfort of IBS. You also must take the responsibility to learn something about those drugs—beyond what they look like and when you need to take them.

Discuss the following questions with your physician:

- What medication are you taking and why?

Be sure you know the medical name for the drug. Have the doctor write it down for you, spelling it phonetically if necessary, so you can pronounce it correctly.

Ask what the particular medication is supposed to do and what symptoms it is supposed to help.

Check to see if you can use a generic substitute or if you are to get the specific drug prescribed. In many states, pharmacies are required to offer the generic substitute if it is cheaper, yet many doctors prefer one particular brand for a good reason. Be sure you know your physician's wishes before you leave the office.

- What are the drug's side effects?

Every medication has its own side effects. You should know them if only to reassure yourself nothing's wrong if your mouth suddenly gets dry or you feel unusually sleepy. By knowing the side effects, you also can help your doctor know if the drug is contraindicated because of the side effects. If you must use a car or heavy machinery in your work, for instance, a drug that makes you sleepy or slows reaction time could be dangerous.

This is also the time, if you haven't done so already, to be sure that you tell your doctor every other medication you are taking—both prescription and over-the-counter. Drugs often interact and mixing the wrong drugs could result in unpleasant side effects. If you can't remember the names of everything you're taking, put all of the bottles in a bag and bring them in to your doctor.

- Do you really need medication?

Sometimes you have to be the best judge of that. A doctor doesn't really know how much pain you feel as pain is a very subjective thing. Ask a number of women who have practiced natural childbirth. Some will tell you it "wasn't too bad." Others will say it "hurt a lot." Who's right? All of them.

Doctors also are only human. They don't like to see people suffer. Sometimes they'll reach for their prescription pad because they know you expect them to prescribe something to make you "feel better." Sometimes they reach for it because they also feel frustrated—as you do—when you don't feel better.

Don't suffer needlessly when there are drugs that can alleviate some of the pain—but also, don't ask for medication unless you really feel that you need it. Sometimes you have to be the judge of just when that point is reached.

Remember that sometimes drugs have a "placebo effect." That means we often feel better just because we're taking something—anything. Studies have shown that the "something" doesn't always have to be actual medication, either. Patients have reported feeling better when the drug taken was just a sugar pill. It doesn't mean they were faking about their pain, either. It only shows the tremendous power our mind has over our body.

Never borrow medicines

Although there are a variety of medications available to help relieve pain, it's unlikely that your doctor will treat your pain with codeine or morphine-based products. In addition to these drugs being potentially addictive, they also aggravate constipation.

Never, never use someone else's painkilling medicine to treat yourself. All medicines have side effects and borrowing a friend's pain medicine, especially if it contains codeine, may result in more pain and discomfort for you in the long run. Also, the dosage prescribed for a friend may be totally wrong for you. Don't try to play doctor. When you self-medicate, you have a fool for a doctor.

Is drug therapy effective with IBS?

There is still much controversy over how effective drug therapy really is with irritable bowel syndrome. One of the major causes of this confusion is that IBS is a chronic disorder, characterized by remission and recurrence. It suddenly goes into remission for no apparent reason, leaving you and the doctor wondering just what it was you both did that made it go away. But before either of you can pat yourself on the back for discovering some new and marvelous treatment for IBS, chances are it will return.

The severity of the symptoms may vary from time to time, but the nature and character of the symptoms remain constant in any one patient.[3] "As a consequence," wrote Dr. John T. Sessions, professor of medicine at the University of North Carolina in Chapel Hill, "the physician must content himself with a therapeutic result somewhat short of complete and lasting remission, in which the treatment should never be more dangerous than the disease."[4]

For this reason, try to understand and be patient if your doctor seems hesitant to prescribe medication for you. At this point, most experts seem to feel that the majority of IBS sufferers can be helped without drugs. Scientists are developing new drugs that would act only on the intestinal nerves and not affect the rest of the body, according to Dr. Michael Gershon of Columbia University, but at this writing, nothing has as yet been perfected.

This is all the more reason why you need to feel comfortable and confident with your physician and have open lines of communication. It's why you need to work together on finding relief from IBS without drugs whenever possible.

Perhaps one day soon a new drug will be found that will target and soothe the overactive intestinal nervous system in all patients and with a minimum of side effects. But until that time, you and your doctor must work hand in hand, through trial and error, to find those approaches that work specifically for you.

Until that time, practice your relaxation techniques and other forms of positive action so you can reduce the effects of negative stress on your body. Each day, expect to feel good and try to focus on well-being, rather than on your symptoms, and look into yourself for relief from IBS, rather than casting an anxious eye to the horizon for some magic pill to appear with the power to make you feel better.

Kids With IBS

"I missed the science fair," the landscape designer told me. "I was twelve, had worked for months on my project—how wind currents affect airplanes—and I got sick the day of the fair. Stomach pains. I always got them."

Now forty, the speaker looked back almost thirty years, and seemed surprised at the memory of how stomach pains disrupted her life even as a young child.

It is estimated that about 2.5 million American children suffer from IBS. In a survey of 1,000 school children, 11 percent were found to have abdominal pain three times in three months, that was severe enough to affect their activity.[1] For many of these children, symptoms seemed to be triggered by stress associated with school problems or stress they felt in relation to their parents' marital problems. As with adults suffering from IBS, there does not seem to be a specific personality type of child who is more prone to this disorder.

According to Dr. Lane France, a Tampa pediatrician, "Many of these children first present symptoms of IBS when they're about ten years old, although they can be as young as five. Their complaint usually is stomach pain, accompanied by cramps that seem worse on eating. Often, their parents think it's 'school phobia' and tend to ignore it. But it's real and needs to be controlled just like irritable bowel syndrome in an adult."

There does tend to be a high familial incidence. According to Dr. Marvin M. Schuster, approximately 75 percent of children with IBS have one or both parents or one or more siblings who suffer from functional gastrointestinal disorders. The two-to-one female predominance found in adults with IBS doesn't hold true with children. In childhood, boys tend to outnumber girls, suggesting that more boys outgrow the syndrome or that females have a later onset, or both.[2]

In children, IBS is often referred to as "RAP," for recurrent abdominal pain. The symptoms tend to drop off in early adolescence and return again in later adolescence.

"It's hard to pinpoint the exact problems," says Dr. William Balistreri, a pediatric gastroenterologist and nutritionist at Children's Hospital Medical Center in Cincinnati. "There's a whole set of common symptoms, but each child is unique. You have to deal with each child as an individual. You can't draw broad references. Parents should never compare notes with their neighbor to see how his or her child was treated."

Children can use detection diaries, too

If your child has IBS, you must quickly accept that it is his or her disorder and he or she must learn to cope with it. You, as a parent, can advise but can't (and shouldn't) hover.

Encourage your youngster to use the detection diaries discussed in Chapter 7. It's a good way for them to try to express what they're feeling. Since stress triggers IBS symptoms in youngsters as well as in adults, the diaries should prove helpful in capturing those elusive mood changes young people experience. In addition, they'll help to document any snacks your child may have eaten at a friend's house, although with younger children it may be more difficult to get them to jot down much detail.

Doctors feel that it's especially important for a child to feel that he or she is actively involved in finding relief for IBS. The diaries can be a useful tool in helping the youngster to feel more responsible.

Through the detection diaries, you and your child can find

recurring patterns that trigger symptoms. Most youngsters are more willing to accept the evidence if they have had a part in writing it down. Once you know what triggers the symptoms, you both can work with the physician to develop ways to find relief. It may be as easy as adding fiber to your child's diet or helping him or her decide on an exercise plan or relaxation program to relieve tension—or it may be more complex, such as letting him or her change schools or join a less competitive sports program.

It's your child's disease

Each physician interviewed said he or she often insisted on seeing the youngster alone, without the parents in the room—especially if the child was an adolescent. It takes time for a doctor to win a young person's trust and to address fears and concerns that the child may hesitate to express.

"Parents shouldn't feel offended when the doctor asks to see the child alone," said Dr. Balistreri. "Sometimes a young person will talk more freely about stresses he or she feels if the parent isn't there.

"Also, IBS is the child's disorder, not the parent's. The youngster must be aware of it each day and act accordingly." As with any other chronic disorder, the patient—child or adult—must understand what triggers problems and learn how to keep those symptoms under control. You can't be with your child every minute of the day, nor should you want to. You and your youngster will feel more confident if the child is aware of what his or her condition is, what triggers it, and how to best cope with its symptoms.

Parents' attitude may affect child

Drs. William E. Whitehead, Marvin M. Schuster, and others feel that illness behavior may be learned by those with IBS in childhood. Studies discussed in earlier chapters revealed that IBS sufferers tended to receive more attention when they were sick as children and that they received gifts and special foods. While parents should never ignore or minimize their child's illness, it is important to refrain from rewarding illness.

Parents also need to be aware that the way they react to their own stress and stomach pains can be copied by their children. This is not to say that the youngsters are "imagining" their pain. Actually, there seems to be growing evidence that the abnormal gut response that causes irritable bowel syndrome runs in families. In addition to this actual weakness of the intestinal nervous system, children also tend to copy their parents' reactions to stress and anxiety. No wonder, as one doctor put it, that "little bellyachers tend to grow up to be big bellyachers."

One of the symptoms physicians look for when taking an adult patient's background for possible diagnosis of IBS is a history of abdominal pain in childhood. In fact, adults who suddenly develop irritable bowel syndrome-type symptoms in their forties or later, without a history of having RAP in childhood, may have something other than IBS.

How to increase fiber

Although some children do have actual food allergies, a major trigger for IBS symptoms in kids is lack of fiber in their diets. In a clinic setting, a youngster often meets with a dietitian to learn how to increase fiber in his diet and how to exclude those foods that cause particular problems.

Dr. William Balistreri suggests you encourage your child to become involved in changing his or her diet by adding fiber. Through the courtesy of the Kellogg Company, I am listing a few "Fiber Fun Recipes for Kids." You might want to read them over with your youngster so he or she can decide which ones to make.

Cooking tips for kids

Cooking is fun and easy. The following guidelines will help you have a successful adventure in the kitchen:

- Wash and dry your hands before preparing a recipe.
- Read the recipe all the way through.
- Gather together all of the ingredients and utensils needed for the recipe.
- When cooking on the range top, turn handles away from you, so they do not catch on anything or turn over.
- To avoid burns use a thick, dry pot holder.
- Wipe up spills immediately.
- When you have completed the recipe, wash and dry utensils and put them away. Wipe counters clean and sweep the floor.

Frosty Yogurt Brananas

5 firm bananas, peeled and halved crosswise
2 containers (6 ounces each, 1½ cups) vanilla yogurt
1½ cups Kellogg's Raisin Bran cereal
10 wooden sticks

1. Place a wooden stick in cut end of each banana. Dip bananas in yogurt to coat. Set aside remaining yogurt.

2. Place bananas on waxed-paper-lined cookie sheet. Freeze one hour or until coating is firm.

3. Dip bananas in remaining yogurt. Roll in Kellogg's Raisin Bran cereal. Return to cookie sheet. Cover with plastic wrap and freeze. Before serving, thaw about 5 minutes.

YIELD: 10 coated Brananas

SERVING: 1 Branana, 100 calories, 2 grams dietary fiber, 1 gram fat.

Giant Raisin Bran Cookie

2 cups Kellogg's Raisin Bran cereal crushed to 1½ cups
1 cup whole wheat flour
1 cup all-purpose flour
1 tsp. baking soda
¾ cup margarine, softened
⅔ cup granulated sugar
½ cup firmly packed brown sugar
2 eggs

1. Stir together Kellogg's Raisin Bran cereal, flours, and soda. Set aside.
2. In large mixing bowl, beat margarine, granulated sugar, and brown sugar until light and fluffy. Add eggs. Beat well. Add flour mixture. Mix thoroughly. Drop by level ¼ cup measure onto ungreased cookie sheet.
3. Bake at 325 degrees for 12 to 14 minutes or until lightly browned.

YIELD: 16 cookies

SERVING: 1 cookie, 250 calories, 2 grams dietary fiber, 12 grams fat.

NOTES: Cookie dough may be frozen. Allow to thaw at room temperature before baking.

You may want to reduce the amount of sugar slightly in this recipe to suit personal taste.

Peanutty Raisin Bran Snacks

½ cup peanut butter
¼ cup honey
½ cup apple juice
3 cups Kellogg's Raisin Bran cereal
¾ cup chopped peanuts (optional)

1. In large mixing bowl, combine peanut butter and honey. Stir in apple juice and Kellogg's Raisin Bran cereal.
2. Measure 1 tablespoon of mixture and shape into a ball.

If desired, roll in chopped nuts. Repeat until all the mixture
is used up. Store in refrigerator. Serve chilled.

YIELD: 25 to 30 snacks

SERVING: 1 snack, 90 calories, 1 gram dietary fiber, 5
grams fat.

NOTE: Peanutty Raisin Bran mixture can be used as a vegetable or fruit spread. Top celery sticks or apple slices with
1 tablespoon of mixture. Sprinkle with chopped peanuts.

Kids' stress can be a pain

There's little doubt that today's youngsters are under tremendous pressures. Psychologist and author David Elkind
refers to them as "hurried children," hurried out of childhood and into a premature adulthood. In his book, *The Hurried Child*, Dr. Elkind writes, "Hurried children are forced
to take on physical, psychological, and social trappings of
adulthood before they are prepared to deal with them. We
dress our children in miniature adult costumes (often with
designer labels), we expose them to gratuitous sex and violence, and we expect them to cope with an increasingly
bewildering social environment—divorce, single parent-
hood, homosexuality."[3]

According to Dr. Lane France, "Probably 85 to 90
percent of the abdominal pain we see in the eight- to fifteen-
year-old age group is triggered by stress." While stress
cannot be completely eliminated from a youngster's life,
coping skills and relaxation techniques discussed in this
section of the book can help to relieve much of the tension.
A child is not too young to learn how to reduce stress.
Success at an early age may make life much more enjoyable
as a youngster gets older.

Be certain that you, as a parent, are not adding to the
stress your youngster experiences. Parental expectations—
expressed or implied—can put a tremendous amount of
pressure on a child.

I have five kids, all of whom have been active in a variety of sports. Through the years that I have attended everything from swim and track meets to soccer, football, baseball, and softball games, I have been amazed (and saddened) by the pressures that sports parents have openly hurled at their kids.

"Strike him out and I'll give you five dollars," shouted one business executive to his twelve-year-old son on the pitcher's mound.

"How could you have missed that tackle?" a mother yelled at her nine-year-old son, who probably didn't weigh as much as his equipment and felt badly enough about his mistake without his mother pointing it out.

"Your sister beat your time," a track mother berated her daughter. "You're going to have to improve if you're ever going to compete with her."

I even heard a swimming coach tell a slightly overweight youngster who had just improved her personal time, although she had not won her meet, "You're too fat. That's why you didn't win."

It's not just in sports that we pressure our kids. In many schools, youngsters burst into tears when they "only" receive a 95 percent on a paper, or get an *A*- rather than an *A*. Parents all over the country maneuver to get their children into the "best" kindergartens so they can get into the "best" prep schools, which of course should prepare them to get into the "best" colleges. Little thought is given to what's "best" for the youngster. Not wanting to appear ungrateful, the children keep silent or express the tension through stomach pain, nausea, and diarrhea.

Help your child by encouraging him or her to express feelings, by listening, by helping him or her to have some unstructured time free from homework, household responsibilities, lessons, or practice—time to relax, to daydream, to just enjoy that brief period called childhood. In a world filled with one-minute responses, it's probably the best gift you can give your youngster.

21

Questions & Answers About IBS

1. What is irritable bowel syndrome?

Irritable bowel syndrome (IBS) is a chronic disorder characterized by altered bowel habits (constipation, diarrhea, or both), stomach pain, and gas with no apparent physical abnormality. Other symptoms may include nausea, vomiting, mucus in the stool, and abdominal bloating.

2. What causes irritable bowel syndrome?

IBS is a movement disorder within the intestine that some people seem to be born with. Many factors, including stress, fatigue, diet, drugs, and hormones, trigger it.

3. Is IBS a serious disease?

It is not a serious disease like cancer or ulcerative colitis, nor does it turn into those diseases. It will not shorten your life expectancy.

4. Can it be cured?

No, IBS cannot be cured. The symptoms may go away for months and even years, but they tend to recur from time to time.

5. How is IBS diagnosed?

Your doctor will make the diagnosis by taking your complete medical history and by conducting a thorough physical examination that probably will include checking your colon visually by using a sigmoidoscope, a small device inserted into the rectum. You'll also have blood taken from your arm for various blood chemistry tests. Stool samples will be tested for parasites and traces of blood too small to be seen with the naked eye. You may have barium contrast X rays. You also may be tested for lactose intolerance. If nothing organic (physical) turns up in all the tests, the doctor will probably make a positive diagnosis of "irritable bowel syndrome." It's called a functional disorder because when the symptoms relate to physiologic changes, there are no structural abnormalities seen on X ray studies.

6. What is "mucous colitis"?

It is an older term for irritable bowel syndrome. It is incorrect, however, because "colitis" refers to an inflammation and there is no inflammation in irritable bowel syndrome. Other terms used for IBS include "spastic colon," "functional colitis," "nervous indigestion," and "irritable colon."

7. What is the colon?

The colon is the large intestine, which extends up from the small intestine, across, and down to the rectum. It is about four to six feet long and acts as a drying tank, removing liquid from waste material before it is expelled as a bowel movement. Food is not digested in the colon; it is digested in the small intestine before reaching the colon.

8. What can my doctor do about my IBS?

Your doctor cannot cure it. He or she can, however:

- identify it
- reassure you that it is not a life-threatening disease
- reassure you that it isn't "all in your head"
- teach you how to reduce stress
- share coping techniques
- tell you how to track down triggers
- help you modify your diet according to *your needs*
- prescribe medications, if needed
- encourage you to lead a normal life

9. How do I know if I have irritable bowel syndrome?

Do not try to diagnose it yourself! Many serious diseases have similar symptoms. You must see a physician who will take your medical history and run the tests described ear-

lier. Only a qualified physician can tell you whether it is
IBS or something else.

10. If I am constipated, is it all right to take a laxative or
stool softener?

Check with your physician. You may not really be constipated. Some people don't have a bowel movement every
day. That may be normal for them. If you miss a day, it
won't hurt you. Laxatives can be habit-forming and make
normal elimination more difficult. Before reaching for a laxative, drink an extra glass or two of water and go walking.
Extra fluids and light exercise often work wonders.

11. Isn't there a special "IBS Diet" that will help me?

Each person must determine his or her own special IBS
diet for specific circumstances. The "Tracking" section of
this book should help you. No one diet is right for every
IBS patient. Food by itself doesn't cause irritable bowel
syndrome. Specific foods can, however, trigger symptoms
under a certain set of circumstances.

12. Can medicines trigger IBS symptoms?

Yes. People with IBS who take laxatives when they think
they are constipated often trigger a siege of diarrhea. Other
medications such as antibiotics, antacids, iron pills, and
even aspirin can cause a recurrence of irritable bowel
syndrome. Always write down everything you take—
prescription or over-the-counter—so you can tell your doctor. Remember that alcohol is a drug, too, and can trigger
IBS symptoms.

13. Is the problem "in my head?"

No, it's in your colon. Stress and emotional tension can,
however, trigger strong movement within the colon. But the
pain is real and it comes from within your intestinal tract.

14. Is lactose intolerance the same thing as irritable bowel
syndrome?

No, although the symptoms are the same. Having lactose
intolerance can *trigger* IBS symptoms, but it also is possible
to have the lactose intolerance without having IBS. People
who have lactose intolerance are unable to properly digest
milk products. An easy way to determine if you have this

problem is to eliminate all milk products from your diet for about two weeks and see if your symptoms disappear.

15. Will eating bran help with constipation?

Most IBS sufferers find that eating bran helps with their constipation. Some people, however, cannot tolerate the extra fiber. Everyone is different and each person must, with the physician's help, determine what works best for him or her.

16. How does irritable bowel syndrome differ from ulcerative colitis?

Both diseases have diarrhea as one of their symptoms, but although IBS is a chronic disease, it is not a serious one in that it is not life threatening. Ulcerative colitis is an inflammation of the lining of the colon with accompanying bleeding, pus, and frequent diarrhea. Whereas people suffering from ulcerative colitis are more prone to cancer of the colon, those with IBS have no greater risk than any other group. That's why you must never try to diagnose yourself but instead get a qualified medical opinion.

17. Is IBS contagious?

No. You can't catch it from someone else. It does, however, seem to run in families, which may mean that the abnormality of the colon is hereditary or that we tend to learn or copy ways of handling stress from our parents.

18. Do children have IBS, too?

Yes. Many children have frequent stomachaches that keep them home from school. The condition is referred to as "RAP," or recurrent abdominal pain. Most adults with IBS report having had stomach pain when they were children.

19. If I have IBS, how can I prevent my children from having it, too?

Since doctors don't really know what causes IBS, it's hard to totally prevent it. You can help minimize the effects, however, by making sure that your children eat a balanced diet with adequate fiber, drink plenty of liquids, preferably water, and learn how to relax when they're feeling tense. Try to minimize discussions about bowel irregularities and don't hover when they're not feeling well. Studies show that many adults with IBS were once children who received undue attention when they were sick.

20. My doctor says I have irritable bowel syndrome. Should I seek another opinion?

It's always safe to get a second opinion. But if that doctor agrees with the diagnosis of IBS, accept it. Don't shop around for yet another doctor. It's not only time-consuming and expensive, but you really don't need more X rays or uncomfortable and invasive tests.

21. What is the most important thing to remember about having IBS?

Accept that although irritable bowel syndrome is chronic (i.e., you don't get cured), it is not a life-threatening disease. It doesn't turn into cancer or ulcerative colitis. Find out what works best for you, follow your doctor's advice, stop worrying about your bowels, and start thinking about how beautiful each day really is.

22

Conclusion

According to Dr. Sidney Cohen of the University of Pennsylvania School of Medicine, "Although the bowel disorder is always present (in patients with IBS), its potential for causing spasm or pain is achieved only through some *inciting factor*, usually diet or emotional stress."[1]

By following the *Relief from IBS* program, you should be able to discover these inciting factors, learning what triggers IBS symptoms in *you*. Armed with this specific information, you can then begin to make those changes in your life which will truly bring you relief from IBS.

Can it work? Dr. Henry J. Tumen of the University of Pennsylvania Graduate Hospital stresses the importance of the patient's self-education and detection by saying, "The patient as an individual is the important factor to be considered in an effort to treat irritable bowel syndrome. It is the education of the individual patient in his own reaction, his responses of life situations, and his ability to cope with these that can bring about successful treatment in irritable colon."[2]

Proper treatment for irritable bowel syndrome is not a simple one-step solution. It requires a great deal of time on your physician's part to slowly piece together the various triggers that affect you in order to prescribe methods of treatment. While it's easy to sit back, expecting your physician to "solve the problem," you must become an active participant. By using what you have learned in *Relief from*

195

IBS, you should be able to take giant strides in helping your physician help you gain relief from irritable bowel syndrome.

Is it effective, this keeping of "detection diaries," practicing relaxation techniques, learning time management skills, and being assertive? Yes. Does it always work? No.

Just recently, I took a long-awaited vacation to London. I really had looked forward to the trip and to visiting friends over there. But I was overtired and under stress from last-minute revisions of plans, and I suffer from flight fright anyway. Before we boarded the plane, some of my familiar IBS symptoms returned.

It was especially frustrating because I've had little discomfort from IBS in the last few years. It also was embarrassing because here I was, writing a book about getting relief from irritable bowel syndrome, and I wasn't feeling much relief.

Then I took my own advice. I began talking to myself, reminding myself that I *had* been free from symptoms for quite some time. I thought about the effects of stress and how it could trigger symptoms. I remembered the comforting sensations I had given myself when I practiced relaxation.

There, in the waiting area of the airport, I closed my eyes and began to concentrate on the black velvet curtain, the image that usually brings me into the relaxation mode. My breathing slowed, my tension level dropped, and I was able to return in my mind to the swing on top of the hill and feel the warmth of the sun as I slowly went back and forth on my imagined swing.

While the relaxation didn't give me total relief for all of my symptoms, it did reduce the severity of the discomfort I had originally felt. I also watched what I ate over the next few days and practiced relaxation daily. I enjoyed my holiday and was reassured that the techniques offered in this book can help give relief to those suffering from irritable bowel syndrome.

Remember that irritable bowel syndrome is a chronic disorder. That means that it won't go away. But the troublesome symptoms do wax and wane. "Most people," concludes Dr. Marvin M. Schuster, "can be helped. A very small proportion can get over their symptoms, and the rest can modify their symptoms."

It is my hope that you have been helped in doing just that through *Relief from IBS*. Good luck.

Suggested Reading

Burkitt, Denis, M.D. *Eat Right—To Stay Healthy and Enjoy Life More*. New York: Arco Publishing, 1979.

Chey, William Y., M.D. *Functional Disorders of the Digestive Tract*. New York: Raven Press, 1983.

Cousins, Norman. *Anatomy of an Illness*. New York: Bantam Books, 1981.

Elkind, David. *All Grown Up & No Place to Go*. Reading, PA: Addison-Wesley Publishing Company, 1984.

Elkind, David. *The Hurried Child—Growing Up Too Fast Too Soon*. Reading, PA: Addison-Wesley Publishing Company, 1981.

Goldberg, Dr. Myron D., and Rubin, Julie. *The Inside Tract*. Washington, D.C.: American Association of Retired Persons, 1986.

Hunter, J.O., M.A., M.D., F.R.C.P., and Jones, Alun V., B.A., M.B., B.Chir. *Food and the Gut*. London: Bailliere Tindall, 1985.

Janowitz, Henry D., M.D. *Your Gut Feelings*. New York: Oxford University Press, 1987.

Plaut, Martin E., M.D. *The Doctor's Guide to You and Your Colon*. New York: Harper & Row, 1982.

Reed, Nicholas W. *Irritable Bowel Syndrome*. London: Grune & Stratton, Ltd., 1985.

Thompson, W. Grant. *The Irritable Gut*. Baltimore: University Park Press, 1979.

Whitehead, William E., and Schuster, Marvin M. *Gastrointestinal Disorders*. Orlando, FL: Academic Press, 1985.

Notes

Chapter 1
1. W. G. Thompson and K. W. Heaton, "Functional bowel disorders in apparently healthy people," *Gastroenterology* 79 (1980): 283–288.

Chapter 3
1. D. A. Drossman, D. W. Powell, and J. T. Sessions, Jr., "The irritable bowel syndrome," *Gastroenterology* 73 (1977): 811–822.
2. A. P. Manning, W. G. Thompson, K. W. Heaton, and A. F. Morris, "Towards positive diagnosis of the irritable bowel," *British Medical Journal* ii (1978): 653.
3. I. G. Hislop, "Childhood deprivation: An antecedent of the irritable bowel syndrome," *Medical Journal of Australia* 1 (9) (1979): 372–374.
4. Ernie Chaney, M.D., "Irritable Bowel Syndrome—A Round Table Sponsored by the Coalition of Digestive Disease Organizations," *Practical Gastroenterology* 8 (4) (July/August 1984): 11.

Chapter 4
1. Hans Selye, *The Stress of Life* (New York: McGraw Hill Book Co., 1976), 418.
2. Nicholas W. Read, *Irritable Bowel Syndrome* (Orlando, FL: Grune & Stratton, Inc., Harcourt Brace Jovanovich, Publishers, 1985), 248.
3. D. A. Drossman, R. S. Sandler, D. C. McKee, and A. J. Lovitz, "Bowel patterns among subjects not seeking health care," *Gastroenterology* 83 (1982): 529–543.
4. Betsy C. Lowman, Ph.D., Douglas A. Drossman, M.D., Elliot M. Cramer, Ph.D., and Daphne C. McKee, Ph.D.,

"Recollection of Childhood Events in Adults with Irritable Bowel Syndrome," *Journal of Clinical Gastroenterology* 9 (3) (1987): 324–330.

5. Walter B. Cannon, "The movement of the intestine studied by means of roentgen rays," *American Journal of Physiology* 6 (1902): 251.

6. T. P. Almy, F. Kern, Jr., and M. Tulin, "Alteration in colonic functions in man under stress: Experimental production of sigmoid spasm in healthy persons," *Gastroenterology* 12 (1949): 425.

7. Thomas Holmes and Richard Rahe, "The Social Readjustment Rating Scale," *Journal of Psychosomatic Research* 11 (1967): 212–218.

8. William E. Whitehead, Ph.D., Bernard T. Engel, Ph.D., and Marvin M. Schuster, M.D., "Irritable Bowel Syndrome," in *Digestive Diseases and Sciences*, New Series Vol. 25, No. 6 (June 1980). Plenum Publishing Corporation.

9. C. M. Bergeron and G. I. Monto, "Personality patterns seen in irritable bowel syndrome patients," *American Journal of Gastroenterology* 80 (1985): 448–451.

Chapter 5
1. N. S. Painter and D. P. Burkitt, "Diverticular diseases of the colon: A deficiency disease of western civilization," *British Medical Journal* 2 (1971): 450.

2. J. O. Hunter, E. Workman, and V. Alun Jones, "The roles of diet in the management of irritable bowel syndrome," in *Topics in Gastroenterology* Vol 12, ed. P. R. Gibson and D. P. Jewel (Oxford: Blackwell Scientific, 1985).

Chapter 6
1. V. Alun Jones and J. O. Hunter, *Doctor, There's Something Wrong with My Guts*, ed. R. E. Pounder (Welwyn Garden City: Smith Kline and French Laboratories, Ltd., 1983), 183–192.

Chapter 7
1. D. A. Drossman, D. W. Powell, and J. T. Sessions, Jr., "The irritable bowel syndrome," *Gastroenterology* 73 (1977): 811–822.

2. W. Grant Thompson, *The Irritable Gut* (Baltimore: University Park Press, 1979), 217.

3. Douglas A. Drossman, M.D., "The Physician and the Patient: Review of the Psychosocial Gastrointestinal Literature

with an Integrated Approach to the Patient," in *Gastrointestinal Disease: Pathophysiology, Diagnosis, Management*, ed. M. H. Sleisenger and J. S. Fordtrain (Philadelphia: W. B. Saunders Company, 1983).

4. Douglas A. Drossman, M.D.; Daphne C. McKee, Ph.D.; Robert S. Sandler, M.D., M.P.H.; C. Madeline Mitchell, M.U.R.P.; Betsy C. Lowman, Ph.D.; Amy L. Burger, M.A.; and Elliot M. Cramer, Ph.D., "Psychosocial Factors in the Irritable Bowel Syndrome: A Multivariate Study of Patients and Nonpatients with IBS," *Gastroenterology* 08:19:54, 1988.

Chapter 8
1. Norman Cousins, *Anatomy of an Illness* (New York: Bantam Books, 1981).
2. Marvin M. Schuster, "Irritable Bowel Syndrome," in *Current Therapy in Gastroenterology and Liver Disease*, 2 (Philadelphia: B.C. Decker, 1986), 345.

Chapter 9
1. G. A. Fava and L. Pavan, "Large bowel disorders. I. Illness configuration and life events," *Psychotherapy and Psychosomatics* 27 (1976–1977): 93–99.
2. R. B. Sandler, D. A. Drossman, H. P. Nathan, and D. C. McKee, "Symptom complaints and health care seeking behavior in subjects with bowel dysfunction," *Gastroenterology* 87 (1984): 314–318.
3. B. D. Pimparkar, "Irritable colon syndrome," *Journal of the Indian Medical Association*, 54 (1970): 95–103.

Chapter 11
1. William Shakespeare, *Hamlet*, act 2, sc. 2.

Chapter 12
1. William E. Whitehead and Marvin M. Schuster, *Gastrointestinal Disorders* (Orlando, FL: Academic Press, 1985), 200.
2. Douglas A. Drossman, "Patients with Psychogenic Abdominal Pain: Six Years' Observation in the Medical Setting," *American Journal of Psychiatry* 139 (December 1982): 1555.

Chapter 13
1. E. D. Jacobson, "Spastic esophagus and mucous colitis: Etiology and treatment by progressive relaxation," *Archives of Internal Medicine* 39 (1987): 433–445.

Chapter 14
1. C. Madeline Mitchell and Douglas A. Drossman, "The Irritable Bowel Syndrome: Understanding and Treating a Biopsychosocial Illness Disorder," *Annals of Behavioral Medicine* 9 (3) (1987): 17.
2. F. Bueno-Miranda, M. Cerulli, and M. M. Schuster, "Operant conditioning of the colonic motility in the irritable bowel syndrome," *Gastroenterology* 70 (5) (1976): 867.
3. W. E. Whitehead, A. S. Fedoravicius, B. Blackwell, and S. Wooley, "A behavioral conceptualization of psychosomatic illness: Psychosomatic symptoms as learned responses," in *Behavioral Approaches to Medicine*, ed. J. S. McNamara (New York: Plenum, 1979), 65–99.

Chapter 17
1. Chesley Hines, Jr., M.D., from symposium, "Dietary Fiber: New Investigations and Clinical Perspectives," held May 2, 1987, and sponsored by Tufts University School of Nutrition. From a speech titled, "Guidelines for the Practitioner: Dietary Fiber, Supplements, and Patient Management."
2. P. A. Cann, N. W. Read, and C. D. Holdsworth, "What is the benefit of coarse wheat bran in patients with irritable bowel syndrome?" *Gut* 25 (1984): 168.
3. J. O. Hunter and V. Alun Jones, *Food and the Gut* (Eastbourne, East Sussex: Bailliere Tindall, 1985), 210.
4. Marvin M. Schuster, M.D., "What to Feed the Patient with Irritable Bowel Syndrome," *Practical Gastroenterology* (1987) (reprint, Shugar Publishing, Inc.).

Chapter 18
1. S. H. Wright, W. J. Snape, Jr., et al., "Effect of dietary components on the gastrocolic response," *American Journal of Psychology* 283 (3) (1980): G228–232.

Chapter 19
1. Douglas A. Drossman, medical seminar in New York, January 19, 1988.
2. K. W. Somerville, C. R. Richmond, and G. D. Bell, "De-

layed release peppermint oil capsules (Colpermin) for the spastic colon syndrome: A pharmacokinetic study," *British Journal of Clinical Pharmacology* 18 (1984): 638–640.
3. S. L. Waller and J. J. Misiewicz, "Prognosis in the irritable bowel syndrome: A prospective study," *Lancet* 2 (1969): 753–756.
4. John T. Sessions, "The Irritable Bowel Syndrome: Diagnosis, Treatment, and Prognosis," *Gastroenterology* 73 (1977): 811–822.

Chapter 20
1. J. Apley and N. Nash, "Recurrent abdominal pain: A field survey of 1000 school children," *Archives of Disease in Childhood* 33 (1958): 165–170.
2. M. Silverberg and F. Daum, "IBS in children and adolescents," *Practical Gastroenterology* 2 (1979): 25.
3. David Elkind, *The Hurried Child: Growing Up Too Fast Too Soon* (Reading, PA: Addison Wesley Publishing Company, 1981).

Chapter 22
1. Sidney Cohen, M.D., "On IBS: A Most Benign Misery," *Executive Health Report* (February 1985).
2. Henry J. Tumen, "The Treatment of Irritable Colon," in *Functional Disorders of the Digestive Tract*, ed. William Y. Chey (New York: Raven Press, 1983), 332.

INDEX

About the Author

Elaine Fantle Shimberg has written on a variety of medical subjects and is a member of both the American Medical Writer's Association and the American Society of Journalists and Authors. Ms. Shimberg resides with her family in Tampa, Florida.

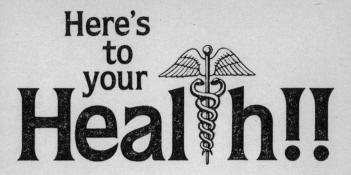